Marketing and General Practice

Marketing and General Practice

COLIN GILLIGAN
Professor of Marketing

ROBIN LOWE
Senior Lecturer in Marketing

RADCLIFFE MEDICAL PRESS • OXFORD and NEW YORK

© 1994 Radcliffe Medical Press Ltd.
18 Marcham Road, Abingdon, Oxon OX14 1AA, UK

Radcliffe Medical Press, Inc
141 Fifth Avenue, New York, NY 10010, USA

Reprinted 1995

British Library Cataloguing in Publication Data
A catalogue record for this book is available from the British Library

ISBN 1 85775 027 6

Typset by AMA Graphics Ltd., Preston
Printed and bound in Great Britain by
Biddles Ltd., Guildford and King's Lynn

The authors

Colin Gilligan is Professor of Marketing at Sheffield Business School. He is the author of books on advertizing, business decision making, international marketing and, most recently, strategic marketing management. Over the past 10 years, he has acted as a consultant to a wide variety of organizations, including numerous medical practices.

Robin Lowe is Senior Lecturer in Marketing and Head of the Small Business Research Unit at Sheffield Business School. He has had 25 years experience in management and consultancy in both large and small organizations, particularly in the healthcare sector.

Preface

This short book, which is based upon our experiences of working with a wide variety of practices over the past three years, is designed to provide general practitioners with a clear understanding of the nature of marketing and of the ways in which it might possibly contribute to the effective management of their practices in the mid to late 1990s. In designing the book, we have concentrated on producing short(ish) chapters that are capable not only of being digested easily in one sitting but which, through a series of questions and checklists, may readily be applied to individual practices.

In working your way through the book and its various checklists, you should not, however, focus just upon the individual questions that we pose, but should also spend time trying to identify the underlying picture that emerges. Is it the case, for example, that the partners *really* recognize the nature and significance of the changes taking place and have a strategy for coming to terms with them, or is it that there is a lack of any real strategy, with the partners being wedded to past and increasingly inappropriate approaches?

Having reached the end of the book, you should have a far clearer idea not only of the nature and purpose of marketing, but also of the ways in which the practice can best make use of marketing techniques and, by means of a series of action plans, move ahead to make the most of the undoubted opportunities that exist. To help illustrate the applications of some of the concepts introduced, we have included a brief case study at the end of the book, The Psalter Lane Surgery. Although this case is based very heavily upon one particular practice, we have introduced elements from other practices and, in the finest traditions of 1930's cinema industry, changed the names to protect the innocent (and the guilty!).

If you feel sufficiently inspired to go further in your study of marketing, there are two books which you might find useful: *Strategic Marketing Management: planning, implementation and control* by Professors Dick Wilson & Colin Gilligan (published by Butterworth Heinemann) and *Marketing for Health Care Organisations* by Philip Kotler and Roberta Clarke (published by Prentice Hall).

Colin Gilligan

Robin Lowe

August 1994

Dedication

This book is dedicated to the authors' wives, Rosie and Sylvia, and children, Ben Gilligan and Jonathan and Catherine Lowe, for their support; and to the GPs whose marketing programme, it is hoped, will benefit from the book.

Contents

The challenges facing general practice

Having read this chapter, you should:

- understand the nature and significance of the challenges facing general practice;

- have a better understanding of the factors that contribute to good management practice;

- have gained an insight into the quality of the management within your practice.

The need for a more conscious, focused and proactive approach to the management of general practice has increased substantially over the last few years. Because of this, we begin not by plunging straight into a detailed discussion of the marketing process, but by taking a broader approach in which we highlight some of the challenges that GPs are now having to face. Having done this, we move on to examine some of the characteristics of good and bad management practice. It is then against this background that in subsequent chapters we turn our attention to the question of marketing and how it might best contribute to the management of general practice in the mid to late 1990s.

THE CHALLENGES FACING GPs

As a first step, refer to Box 1.1 and begin by identifying the six principal challenges which you believe your practice is likely to face and have to come to terms with

Box 1.1:   The short and long term challenges faced by the practice

The principal challenges that the practice is likely to face are:

Short term

1 . . . .

2 . . . .

3 . . . .

4 . . . .

5 . . . .

6 . . . .

Long term

1 . . . .

2 . . . .

3 . . . .

4 . . . .

5 . . . .

6 . . . .

in the short (that is the next twelve to eighteen months) and then the longer term.

Although the *particular* challenges faced will vary – possibly significantly from one practice to another – our work with almost 50 different practices over the past three years has identified a number of areas which practice managers and doctors alike see as being of special concern. These include:

- greater accountability to patients;

- greater accountability to a seemingly ever more demanding FHSA;

- increased patient choice and a greater willingness of patients to move from one practice to another;

- financial pressures;

- issues relating to fundholding;

- a need for far more attention to be paid to the practice's image;

- a need to decide more clearly upon the focus of the practice and, in particular, which clinics to offer;

- the need for many practices to develop more effective, and possibly more mature relationships with suppliers of hospital services;

- increased intervention from the government;

- a need for more and better staff training and motivation;

- the problem of crumbling and increasingly bureaucratic health authorities;

- computerization and data protection;

- an increase in the volume of paper;

- increased patient expectations and aggression;

- the need for a more competitive philosophy;

- issues surrounding accommodation;

- setting, being set and meeting targets;

- the need for better internal and external communication;

- managing the relationship between the doctors and the other members of the practice.

Although this is not by any means an exhaustive list and the relative importance of each of the points is likely to vary greatly from one practice to another, it highlights the nature and breadth of the sorts of changes and challenges that are currently facing general practice and which the practice's management team needs to come to terms with. From your viewpoint as a doctor, the question that must, of course, be considered is how each of these challenges can best be managed. However, before trying to answer this, consider the questions at the top of the next page and then ask yourself what picture is beginning to emerge. Is it the case, for example, that the practice not only recognizes the nature and significance of the challenges and has begun to come to terms with them by means of a deliberate approach to management, or is it that there is a general reluctance to change old habits and working practices?

- To what extent have these challenges been given *explicit* recognition in the practice?

- What *specific* plans exist to deal with them?

- Has the *responsibility* for dealing with these challenges been allocated?

THE CHARACTERISTICS OF GOOD AND BAD MANAGEMENT

Over the past 50 years, a considerable amount has been written about the characteristics of good and bad management. One result of this is that a series of increasingly specific guidelines exist. However, before looking at some of these, consider the question in Box 1.2.

The reality, of course, is that it is difficult (if not impossible) to identify the six or ten characteristics of good and bad management which will apply equally to every type and size of organization. What we can do, however, is to identify the sorts of areas to which every organization, be it a medical practice or a multinational manufacturer of foodstuffs or cars, needs to give serious consideration. Included within these are:

Box 1.2:   The characteristics of good and bad management

What do you consider to be the six principal characteristics of good and bad management?

Good management   Bad management

1 . . . .   1 . . . .

2 . . . .   2 . . . .

3 . . . .   3 . . . .

4 . . . .   4 . . . .

5 . . . .   5 . . . .

6 . . . .   6 . . . .

- a statement of the organization's mission and overall purpose;

- the development of strong and positive values which are understood and adhered to by all staff;

- the development of clear and realistic objectives which, where possible, are agreed as the result of discussion amongst the staff, so that there is a sense of shared ownership of the goals and strategy;

- strong and unambiguous patterns of communication which allow information to go upwards, downwards and sideways quickly without being distorted;

- a sense of teamwork;

- a clear allocation of responsibilities;

- a sustained effort to motivate staff at *all* levels;

- systems for monitoring progress, feeding back the results, and taking corrective action on the basis of this;

- a climate which encourages rather than suppresses ideas;

- a management philosophy which encourages a degree of independence amongst staff;

- a management philosophy which encourages staff to get things done correctly on time;

- a recognition of staff needs (both personal and organizational);

and, most importantly of all

- an open and consistent management style, since one of the most widely accepted findings in management research is that one of the prime demotivators of staff is a lack of consistency in management style. Where the approach adopted fluctuates between autocratic, democratic and laissez-faire styles, seemingly depending upon how the wind is blowing, staff end up being confused and as a result, tend to focus upon a series of increasingly short-term issues.

Taking each of these areas in turn, you need firstly to compare them with the list of the characteristics of good management that you have developed for

Box 1.3:   Scoring the quality of your practice's management

On a scale of 1–5 (1 = very poor, 5 = very good), how does your practice score on each of the following dimensions of good management?

                                                                    Score 1–5

1.   The clarity of the mission and overall purpose   ____
2.   Strong and positive values   ____
3.   The clarity and appropriateness of the objectives   ____
4.   The effectiveness of communications patterns   ____
5.   Levels of teamworking   ____
6.   Allocation of responsibilities   ____
7.   Levels of motivation   ____
8.   Use of monitoring systems   ____
9.   The encouragement of ideas   ____
10. Staff independence   ____
11. Getting things done correctly and on time   ____
12. The recognition of staff needs   ____
13. The management style   ____

                                                          Total   ____

The scoring process
With a total score of 29 or less, the practice is likely to lack direction and control with the result that motivation and morale almost inevitably will be low.

With a score of 30–44 there is scope for considerable improvement.

With a score of 45–54, there is scope for some improvement, but you will probably have to work hard at this. There is certainly no room for complacency.

With a score of 55–65, you need to ask yourself just how honest you have been in your scoring process. If having done this, you still feel the score is justified, again you need to guard against complacency to ensure that your currently very high standards do not slip.

Box 1.2 and then, secondly, consider how well (or how badly) your practice scores; the framework for this appears in Box 1.3.

These sorts of ideas have also been brought together in the powerful and widely used 7S model which was developed in the United States in the 1980s by the management consultants, McKinsey; this is illustrated in Figure 1.1.

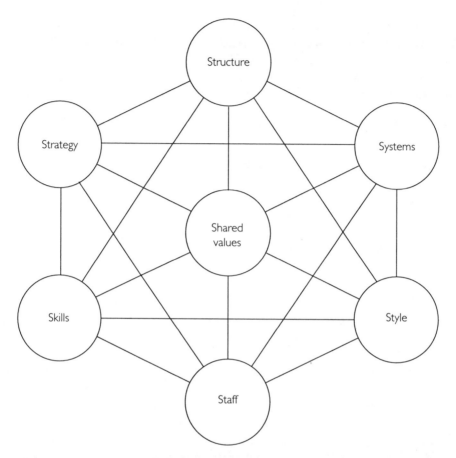

Figure 1.1:   The McKinsey 7S framework

The importance of the first three elements – strategy, structure and systems – has long been recognized and are considered to be the *hardware* of successful management. The other four – style, staff, skills and shared values – represent the *software*.

For much of the past 50 years, management thinking has been firmly based on the need to ensure that the hardware elements exist. Thus, a successful organization, it has been argued, builds a *strategy* to achieve its goals, develops an appropriate organizational *structure*, and then equips the organization with the sorts of information, planning, control and reward *systems* needed to ensure that the job gets done. The starting point in this is therefore that a strategy is needed before decisions on structure and systems are made.

The importance of the four software elements has been given substantially increased recognition over the past decade largely as the result of research work in what came to be labelled 'excellent' companies; these were organizations which achieved substantially better levels of performance and customer satisfaction than their competitors. The characteristics of these four elements are:

Style:
Employees share a broadly common way of thinking and behaving. In organizations such as Marks & Spencer and McDonald's, for example, all employees are taught to treat customers in a particular and caring way.

Skills:
Employees are fully trained in the sorts of skills that are needed to carry out the tasks associated with the strategy.

Staff:
The people recruited are capable, well-trained, and given the jobs which allow them to make the best use of their talents.

Shared values:
The employees share the same values, understand where the organization is going and what it stands for.

Given these comments, you need to consider how your practice performs in relation to each of these dimensions; the framework for this appears in Box 1.4 opposite.

With regard to the software elements, arguably the most important single factor is the idea of shared values. There are several ways in which shared values can be developed within a practice, but most obviously by means of an open management style which encourages discussion, communication, and a sense of common purpose amongst all staff, but particularly the management team. In the case of general practice, this will typically include the doctors and the practice managers. Between you, you should therefore aim for a statement which brings together the core values of the organization (for example, a fundamental commitment to quality and excellence), and a vision of the sort of practice that as a team you are trying to create.

Box 1.4:   The application of the McKinsey 7S framework to your practice

1. Looking at each of the elements of the 7S framework, on a scale of 1–5 (1 = very poor, 5 = very good), how does your practice score?

	Score 1–5
Strategy	____
Structure	____
Systems	____
Style	____
Skills	____
Staff	____
Shared values	____
Total	**__**

2. Where are the areas of the greatest apparent weakness?

3. What scope exists for improvement?

4. What are you planning to do about this?

SUMMARY

Within this chapter we have identified a series of the challenges that general practice is currently having to face, and highlighted some of the principal characteristics of good and bad management. In the light of your answers to the questions that we have posed, consider, therefore, the following:

1. What underlying picture of the practice emerges?

2. What do you feel are the principal causes of this picture, be it good or bad?

3. What sorts of answers do you feel that staff within the practice might have given to the questions posed in the Boxes? To what extent do these differ from your own views?

So what is marketing?

Having read this chapter, you should:

- understand the marketing concept and how it can be applied within general practice;

- appreciate the significance of different stakeholder groups and the need to take their expectations into account;

- understand the structure of the marketing process.

Given the nature of our comments in Chapter one, it is apparent that as general practice faces some of its biggest changes and challenges of the post-war period, the need for tighter, more professional and forward-looking management is greater than ever before. In many cases this has meant a substantial rethink of how practices are run and how a variety of the managerial tools and techniques that previously were seen to be the prerogative of manufacturers in the private sector, and hence of little real relevance to doctors, might now possibly contribute to the better and more effective management of general practice. Prominent amongst these is the whole area of marketing. In many cases, however, there appears still to be a fundamental misunderstanding amongst doctors of precisely what marketing involves and how it might most realistically contribute either to the effective day-to-day management of the practice, or indeed to its longer term development.

Within this chapter, we concentrate on overcoming some of the more common preconceptions and misconceptions of marketing that we have encountered in a variety of practices, and move towards developing a framework which should go some way towards establishing a stronger – and far more effective – marketing and patient–centred orientation within the practice.

WHAT MARKETING IS AND WHAT MARKETING IS NOT

Consider the four statements in Box 2.1 to see which corresponds most closely with your view of marketing.

Box 2.1:   Marketing is . . .

1.   . . . the same as advertizing

2.   . . . something which is used solely by large firms and of little or no real relevance to general practice

3.   . . . manipulative and is really a hard sell in disguise

4.   . . . an approach to management which applies to all types of organization, since it puts the customer (in the case of general practice this is, of course, the patient) at the very centre of the operation (no pun intended) and directs resources in such way that the customer achieves a high level of satisfaction in a cost effective manner.

Those of you who answered 'yes' to any, or indeed all, of the first three should go to the bottom of the class. Those who agreed with number four get top marks.

So what then is wrong with the first three statements? We can illustrate the limitations of the first by focusing upon examples of large organizations whose activities you will undoubtedly be familiar with and which have developed a strong reputation for consistently effective marketing and high levels of customer satisfaction. When members of the public are asked to identify three or four examples of the sorts of organizations which they consider to be good at marketing, the same names almost invariably crop up. Prominent amongst these are Coca Cola, McDonald's, Marks & Spencer and Body Shop. In the case of Coca Cola and McDonald's, both companies concentrate upon using substantial amounts of advertizing to communicate clear and simple messages 'Things go better with Coke' and 'There's nothing quite like a McDonald's' which are understood and seemingly meaningful to customers across the world. They market consistently reliable products and provide levels of service which rarely disappoint. Marks & Spencer, by contrast, has achieved a similarly strong position with little or no advertizing, whilst Body Shop is successful despite spending very little on advertizing, packaging or indeed store layout. Marketing and advertizing are not, therefore, one and the same thing. Rather, advertizing is just one of the marketing tools available.

On a smaller scale, think about your favourite restaurant. Although at first sight it might appear that it does not need marketing to make it successful, look more closely on your next visit at how they operate. Almost inevitably it will have built a clear reputation as, for example, the best Italian, Indian or Chinese restaurant in town. The appearance and decor will project a clear image, the staff will be friendly and the food and drinks will have been selected to meet the demands and expectations of customers who will be made to feel comfortable in these surroundings. To create a successful restaurant, every aspect will have been planned well in advance, reflecting the owner's and manager's beliefs about what the customers they wish to attract will want. However, their task does not end there as they will constantly be trying to improve things and make sure that every aspect of the restaurant is just right. So marketing can, but does not need to depend on advertizing, and is capable of making just as important a contribution to the success of small, as well as to large organizations.

The third common misconception is that marketing is almost invariably manipulative and is selling in disguise; timeshare holiday companies are a notorious example of this. In the long term, however, customer satisfaction cannot be built on manipulation or on false promises. We may fall for it the first time, but only rarely a second time. In the case of timeshare, most members of the public, and not just those who have fallen foul of the timeshare touts, are now only too aware of the typically exaggerated offers that they make and are suspicious of almost *any* offer that is made, regardless of how attractive it appears. The unfortunate result of this has, of course, been that the reputable companies in the industry (and yes, they do exist) which offer a worthwhile product have been affected as well. Because of this, the opportunity for the market to be developed to its full potential has been lost (probably forever) not necessarily because of any failure of the product or service offered, but because of the unacceptably high pressure selling techniques that have been used.

Given these examples, we should be in a far clearer position to identify what marketing in its true sense means and what it involves. Although it is difficult to list *all* of the activities that are normally covered by marketing, the most important can be identified as:

1. Monitoring the external environment with a view to identifying opportunities and threats;

2. Contributing to the discussion about the nature and direction that the organization should pursue;

3. Determining the range of products or services that should be offered;

4. Influencing the levels of customer/patient satisfaction that are to be aimed for;

5. Deciding upon the image that is to be projected;

6. Managing the elements of the marketing mix on a day-to-day basis (the nature of the mix is discussed in figures 2.2, 2.3 and, in detail, in chapter 9);

7. Developing and implementing a system of feedback and control that is capable of providing a clear picture of just how well the practice is performing.

It follows from this that the essence of good marketing involves both a strong *external* and a clear *internal* orientation. External in that we are concerned with building a clear picture of what is happening, and likely to happen, outside the practice so that we might identify and capitalize upon the opportunities that exist, and internal in terms of making sure that what we offer and intend doing is feasible and that the staff understand and are fully committed to this.

DEFINITIONS OF MARKETING

It should be apparent from what has been said so far that marketing is a much more complex activity than simply selling or advertizing the product or service that the organization, be it Marks & Spencer or a doctor's practice, has decided to provide, something which is reflected in the numerous definitions of marketing that exist. Box 2.2 shows just a small selection of these.

THE SIGNIFICANCE OF STAKEHOLDERS

Although in general practice the main strand of any definition of marketing that we use might be translated into *meeting patients' needs*, there is a strong case for arguing that this is too simplistic, since if the practice is to be successful, account needs to be taken not just of patients' needs and expectations, but also those of a variety of other stakeholders (a stakeholder is any individual or group

Box 2.2: Definitions of marketing

- Marketing is the management process for identifying, anticipating and satis-fying customers' requirements (in the case of a commercial organization, we would add the word 'profitably' at the end of the sentence).

- Marketing is the central dimension of any business. It is the whole business seen from the point of view of its final result, that is from the customers' point of view.

- Marketing is all about customer satisfaction and moving heaven and earth to achieve this more effectively than other organizations.

- The marketing concept represents an 'outside-in' view of the organization, in that a deliberate attempt is made to look at the organization and its products/services from the viewpoint of the customer. In doing this, greater emphasis is placed upon meeting customers' needs, selling benefits, achieving higher levels of internal co-ordination and generally achieving a far better match between customers' needs and what the organization offers.

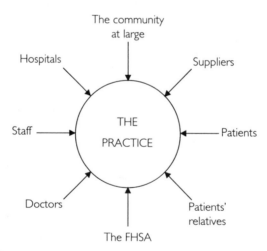

Figure 2.1: The practice's stakeholders

which has an interest in how the practice operates); these are illustrated in Figure 2.1.

Each stakeholder approaches an organization with certain expectations and it is the extent to which these expectations are satisfied that is the true measure of organizational effectiveness. Recognizing this, turn to Box 2.3 and identify, in as much detail as possible, the nature of each of your stakeholder's expectations and then the scope for conflict that exists between the different types of stakeholder.

Box 2.3:   Stakeholders' expectations of our practice

Patients . . . .

Patients' relatives . . . .

Suppliers . . . .

The FHSA . . . .

Partners . . . .

Staff . . . .

Hospitals . . . .

The community at large . . . .

Scope for conflict between these expectations exists in the following areas:

-

-

-

-

Overall, how well do you feel that you manage any conflict that emerges?

What else might you do?

THE TWO LEVELS OF MARKETING

If marketing is to make a significant contribution to general practice, it needs to operate at two levels. At its most fundamental, it represents an underlying philosophy of patient satisfaction which should guide everything that the doctors and staff do. On a day to day basis it is concerned with issues such as the specifics of the product or service that is offered, the practice image that is projected, and how and where the product/service is to be presented. The essence of marketing is therefore to get everyone to pull together and work towards the common goal of customer/patient satisfaction. If this is done, and done effectively, the benefits can be considerable and include:

- higher levels of patient satisfaction;

- a far greater likelihood of identifying market opportunities in their early stages;

- a higher level of awareness of those factors that will ultimately prove to be a threat;

- a better sense of direction and co-ordination;

- a greater opportunity for staff to take more responsibility without loss of control;

- higher levels of staff motivation as a result of their greater understanding, involvement, responsibility and commitment.

THE MARKETING PROCESS

In the light of our comments so far, we can identify the three principal strands of a marketing programme :

1. The pressures of the environment (and hence the nature of any opportunities and threats that exist currently and which are likely to emerge in the future);

2. The demands, needs or expectations of patients and how these are likely to change;

3. What the practice is capable of delivering.

It follows from this that the marketing process consists of four stages: analysis; planning; evaluation and implementation; feedback and control. These are illustrated in Figure 2.2 and expanded upon in Box 2.4.

Stage One: Market analysis

In the first of the four stages, we need to concentrate upon developing a clear understanding of the variety of factors outside the practice. These cannot be

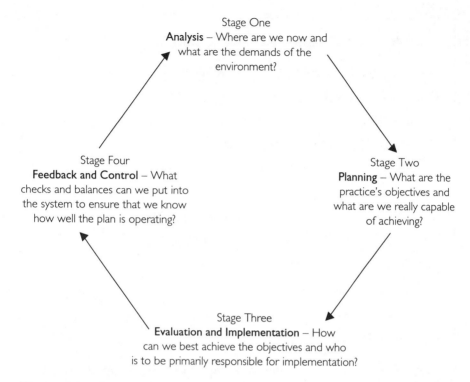

Figure 2.2:   The marketing process

controlled but they determine how the practice operates and are capable of having a very real influence upon its performance, and include the general environment, the changing needs of patients and other stakeholders, and the behaviour of competitors in the healthcare business.

Stage Two: Marketing planning

Against the background of the market analysis, the emphasis needs to shift to planning and, in particular, to the identification of the goals, objectives and standards which the practice will pursue. In doing this, detailed consideration needs to be given to an assessment of the practice's capabilities, since these determine how likely it is that objectives will be met and whether any gaps exist between the practice's aspirations and objectives, and its capabilities (in other words, what you are really capable of delivering). This information can then be brought together in the form of a plan which will be the blueprint for practice development.

Box 2.4:   The four stages of the marketing process

Stage one: Analysis (Where are we now?)

Analysing and understanding:

- the environment;

- patients' and other stakeholders' needs and expectations;

- competition (what other practices are doing and what we can learn from them and improve upon).

Stage Two: Planning (Where do we want to go?)

Planning for action by:

- setting objectives and standards;

- evaluating practice capabilities;

- researching patient needs;

- planning for change.

Stage Three: Evaluation and implementation (How might we get there?)

Implementing the plan by:

- managing the marketing mix;

- marketing the plan internally;

- developing stakeholder relationships.

Stage Four: Feedback and control (How can we check how well the plan is operating?)

Controlling the plan by:

- developing checks and balances;

- monitoring progress;

- taking corrective action.

Stage Three: Evaluation and implementation

Following this, the focus then turns to the question of how to implement the plan. It has long been recognized that the implementation stage is typically the most difficult part of the marketing planning process, since it is only too easy to lose sight of the objectives, to be blown off course by unforeseen events, and to become preoccupied with day-to-day pressures with the result that longer-term issues are ignored. A key element of marketing is therefore concerned with the question of how best to manage the resources that are available in as effective a manner as possible and ensure that the objectives that have been set are achieved. Because the largest and most costly resource in general practice is that of the staff, much of the implementation phase is, of necessity, concerned with mobilizing the staff and other stakeholders, including those who supply the practice with services and products, by making sure that they understand what is fully expected of them and that they contribute fully in the most appropriate way.

But as well as staff, implementation is integrally tied up with how well the marketing mix is managed. Although we discuss the marketing mix in detail in Chapter nine, there are several comments that can usefully be made at this stage. The marketing mix, which consists of the seven elements illustrated in Figures 2.3 and 2.4, and which is sometimes referred to as the 7Ps, represents the marketing man or woman's tool kit. Despite the strict guidelines and controls that exist within the NHS, these elements can be managed in order to shape the profile of the practice that is presented to the world. As such, the appropriateness of the mix (that is, the match between the mix and the demands of the environment) has a direct influence upon the organization's performance.

Stage Four: Feedback and control

Having implemented the marketing plan, attention needs then to be paid to measuring the performance levels that have been achieved, with a view to identifying any need for modification and improvement. There is, therefore, a need to monitor performance under a variety of headings. These might include:

* financial performance – including income, expenditure and profitability;

* doctors' commitments and performance – including work undertaken, external posts, prescribing patterns and personal development;

* staff performance – including turnover, attitudes, motivation, development and training;

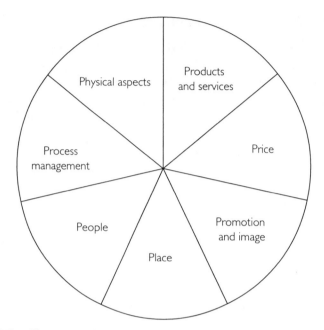

Figure 2.3: The seven elements of the marketing mix

- patient management – including the demand for services, referral patterns, levels of satisfaction with the practice, and list changes;

- premises management – including their suitability and the nature of any improvements made;

- communications management – including the development of the practice's image and the success of any promotional initiatives;

- the development of new services – such as health promotion programmes;

- the introduction of new or modified patient management systems.

However, if this is to be a meaningful activity, it presupposes that the objectives that were set in stage two (marketing planning), have been set clearly and provide a meaningful basis for measurement and comparison over time. This is an issue which we return to in later chapters.

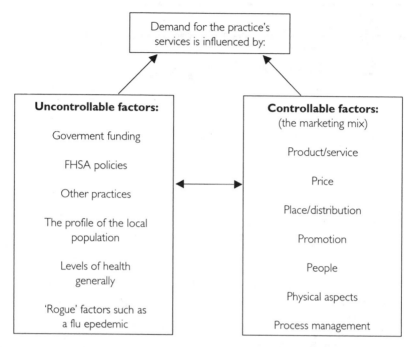

Figure 2.4: The marketing mix and the health service environment

SUMMARY

Within this chapter we have focused upon the nature of marketing and the marketing process as well as the ways in which marketing may be applied to general practice. Although a marketing programme needs to reflect, or at least take account of, the expectations of various stakeholder groups, the primary focus is of how best to achieve a truly patient-centred practice. It is this issue which is developed in the next chapter.

3

Developing the patient-centred practice: the first few steps

Having read this chapter, you should:

- understand the dimensions of a patient-centred practice;

- appreciate the significance of the differences between features and benefits;

- have a clearer insight to the benefits that your practice offers currently and is capable of offering in the future;

- understand in greater detail what it is that your patients want from the practice.

In order to develop a marketing-oriented and truly patient-centred practice, there is an obvious need to understand in detail your market for primary health care and, in particular, the sorts of factors that are likely to lead to higher levels of patient satisfaction. Without this information, any marketing effort will be unfocused and, at best, of only limited value. So what is it that contributes to patient satisfaction? Although most doctors would argue that they have a clear idea of this, it is only the patients themselves who are *really* able to answer the question. Lessons can be learned from the commercial sector which provide some help as to how we might best go about this.

When dealing with a commercial client, we always begin by posing a deceptively simple question: what *benefits* are your customers really looking for? The significance of this is that rarely, if ever, do people buy a product or service for its own sake. Instead, they buy it for the benefits that it provides. Perhaps the most commonly cited example of this is the purchase of a drill which, as the American management guru, Theodore Levitt, pointed out in the 1950s, is bought not for its physical qualities but in order to provide holes.

By the same token, cars such as Porsche, Mercedes, BMW and Jaguar, whether we like to admit it or not, are bought as much for their status, image and prestige as anything else; customers then justify their purchase by highlighting features such as the build quality, the glacier-like depreciation, the pre- and after-sales services, reliability, and so on. Equally, research in the expensive, boxed chocolates market reveals that buying motives are seldom concerned with taste, but are more commonly to do with the perceived value of the product as a gift. In the case of the beer market, the primary buying motives amongst the 18 to 22 year olds have consistently been shown to be concerned not with the beer's taste or strength, but with the images associated with the brand and peer group pressure.

Recognition of this highlights the need for a clear and detailed understanding of the distinctions that exist between features and benefits, since it is this understanding which underpins any attempt to develop a truly patient-centred practice. It is, for example, only too easy to talk about the sorts of things that GPs do (the features) rather than what patients get from it (the benefits). This is likely to be manifested in terms of how a doctor cures a patient's illness; the cure being the *feature*. However, looking at it from the patients' point of view, they go to a GP feeling unwell and wanting to feel better. The extent to which this is achieved is influenced partly by the clinical elements and partly by the series of non-clinical elements, normally referred to as patient service. If these non-clinical features fail to work effectively, the patient may well go away having been cured but feeling unhappy, unconvinced by the treatment and generally dissatisfied.

COMING TO TERMS WITH THE BENEFITS

In order to understand more fully the sorts of benefits that the practice offers currently, you need to begin by looking at features from the patient's viewpoint. There are several ways of doing this, although perhaps the most useful is by focusing in turn upon each of the seven principal elements of the marketing mix identified in Chapter two (see pages 19–21). Here we can illustrate the features/benefit distinction by focusing upon just one of these dimensions, that of the product or service.

The cornerstone of any marketing programme is the nature of the product or service offered, since virtually all other marketing elements and decisions are directly influenced by this. In the case of general practice, the product/service is the collection of benefits that the patient desires. At the core of this 'product' are the clinical services where the traditional values of medical excellence, quality and skill are paramount; examples of those that are typically offered appear in Box 3.1.

Box 3.1:   The core clinical services

- personal medical care

- family planning services

- maternity services

- child health care

- immunizations

- health promotion programmes

- well man/woman programmes

- 24-hour cover

- emergency home visits

- counselling

Surrounding these core clinical services are the various non-clinical support services, including the appointments system, the receptionists, the waiting area, and the manner of the consultation itself; these are illustrated in Figure 3.1.

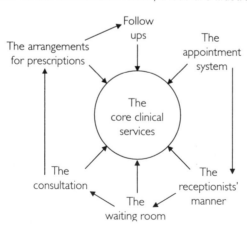

Figure 3.1:   The product/service and the surrounding support mechanisms

Although the question of what benefits the practice offers currently and what it is capable of developing is considered in far greater detail later, a useful first step is to begin by thinking about the specific benefits that patients get from just some of the services you offer. A framework to help you do this appears in Figure 3.2.

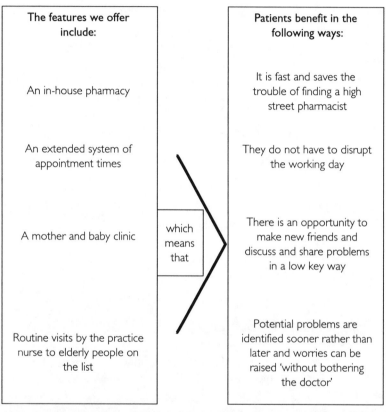

The features we offer include:

An in-house pharmacy

An extended system of appointment times

A mother and baby clinic

Routine visits by the practice nurse to elderly people on the list

which means that

Patients benefit in the following ways:

It is fast and saves the trouble of finding a high street pharmacist

They do not have to disrupt the working day

There is an opportunity to make new friends and discuss and share problems in a low key way

Potential problems are identified sooner rather than later and worries can be raised 'without bothering the doctor'

Figure 3.2:   The features-benefits link

In thinking about the nature and significance of benefits, Herzberg's two-factor theory of motivation can be of some help. The theory distinguishes between *satisfiers* (factors that create satisfaction) and *dissatisfiers* (factors that create dissatisfaction). In the case of a car, for example, the absence of a warranty would be a dissatisfier. The existence of a warranty, however, is not a satisfier since it is not one of the principal reasons for buying the product. Instead, as we suggested earlier, these are more likely to be the car's looks, its performance and the status that the driver feels it lends.

There are several implications of this theory for the marketing of general practice, the two most significant of which are, first, that the seller (that is, the doctor and the practice) needs to be fully aware of the dissatisfiers which, while they will not by themselves sell the product, can easily 'unsell' it. The second implication, which follows logically from this, is that the doctor and the practice staff need to understand in detail the various satisfiers and then concentrate not just upon supplying them, but also giving emphasis to them so that patients are fully aware of them.

It should be apparent from this that achieving a truly patient-centred practice is a potentially difficult task and, for most practices, is likely to involve significant changes in operating practices and culture. Recognizing this, consider the following questions and then move on to the checklist that appears in Box 3.2.

- What are the principal satisfiers and dissatisfiers within the practice?

- What are we doing/can we do to increase the satisfiers and reduce or abolish completely the dissatisfiers?

- What are the obstacles to making the sorts of changes needed in order to achieve a patient-centred practice, how significant are they, and how might we overcome them?

ARE THE APPARENT BENEFITS REALLY BENEFITS?

Perhaps the easiest and most useful way of identifying and assessing the sorts of benefits that patients might get from a service is to apply the 'which means that' and the 'so what' tests. In the case of a practice that is considering an appointments system which offers appointments throughout the day, the implication of the 'which means that' test is that patients are not tied either to the early morning or late afternoon/early evening. The potential benefits for a person who is free during the course of the day are therefore obvious.

However, for a person who, because of work commitments, can only attend the surgery in the evening, the 'so what' test highlights that the change is of no real or direct value (there is, of course, the indirect benefit that because appointments are being spread throughout the day, evening surgery should be that much quieter and an appointment therefore easier to make).

Given this, and appreciating that the benefits to patients are not always as obvious or as significant as might have been hoped or expected at

Box 3.2: How serious are we about patient satisfaction?

1 = Very poor performance;
5 = Average performance but with considerable scope for improvement;
10 = Excellent performance.

**Marks out
of ten**

How good are we at:

1. Measuring levels of patient satisfaction?   ____

2. Using measures of patient satisfaction to change practice policies and operating procedures?   ____

3. Using patient satisfaction measures to
   (a) evaluate staff
   (b) reward staff?   ____

4. Ensuring that *all* practice staff have a clear understanding of our policy on patient service and quality?   ____

5. Setting measurable goals for levels of patient service and quality?   ____

6. Discussing with staff the patients' needs and expectations?   ____

7. Taking formal note of what staff say about patients' needs and expectations and the extent to which they are being met?   ____

8. Doctors setting a good example of the levels of service and quality that are important?   ____

9. Providing opportunities for staff to work together to overcome obstacles to achieve high(er) levels of quality and service?   ____

10. Evaluating how other practices operate and the standards that they are achieving?   ____

11. Evaluating what organizations outside general practice do with a view to learning from them?   ____

12. Implementing a clearly stated and realistic policy on patient service and quality?   ____

                                                   Total (out of 120)   ____

continued over

Box 3.2:   *continued*

The Scoring Process

Each doctor within the practice should work through the twelve questions in order to arrive at a score. The scores should then be aggregated and averaged. The overall measure of commitment to patient service and satisfaction can then be assessed against the following scale:

With a score of 59 or less, questions can be asked about the practice's commitment to patient service. Fundamental changes are needed, both in the practice philosophy and organizational structure.

With a score of between 60–79, there is again scope for improvement.

With a score of between 80–99, scope for improvement still exists, although this is likely to be in terms of a series of small changes and modifications rather than anything more fundamental.

With a score of 100 or more, care needs to taken that doctors and staff maintain the standards being achieved and that complacency does not creep in.

first sight, Figure 3.3 can be used to identify – and, more importantly, assess – the real benefits of any features that you offer currently, or are thinking of developing.

WHAT DO PATIENTS REALLY WANT FROM THEIR DOCTORS?

Over the years, various studies have been conducted in order to find out what patients really want from their doctors. Perhaps the most useful of these was carried out in 1989 by 'Which?' magazine, in which 2,000 patients from across the country and registered with a variety of types of practice were surveyed.

The general pattern of results highlighted the importance of doctor-patient communication and how poor this frequently turns out to be. Although to a large degree these results were broadly predictable, they illustrate the extent to which either doctors have failed to respond to the sorts of comments and criticisms that have been made with increasing frequency over the past twenty years, or to the depth of patient dissatisfaction. Thus:

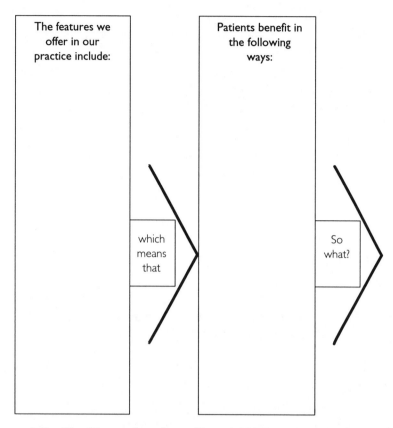

Figure 3.3:   The features, benefits and 'so what' link

- 91% of the respondents felt that their doctor spends too little time explaining the nature, causes and significance of their illness;

- 89% wanted their doctor to spend more time listening;

- 84% of patients wanted more detailed information on hospitals and what was involved with the in-patient and out-patient services to which they were being referred;

- 82% wanted the doctor to spend more time explaining what drugs were being prescribed, how well and how quickly they might be expected to work, and the nature of any possible side-effects;

- 80% wanted the reception staff to be more helpful, understanding and courteous.

There are several issues that emerge from these findings, the three most significant of which are that a remarkably high proportion of patients believe that doctors do not really listen enough, explain things fully, or spend sufficient time on the consultation. A comparison across Europe of how much consultation time is spent with the patient paints an interesting picture; doctors in France spend an average of twenty minutes with each patient, eighteen minutes in Germany, twelve in Italy, and just six in Britain. Although the obvious reaction to this, and indeed the one that we have encountered on numerous occasions in our work with GPs, is that the time is simply not there, this response misses the significance of the point being raised and of course runs counter to the idea of the patient-centred practice.

MOVING AHEAD

Given the nature of these comments, the question of how the truly patient-centred practice might be developed needs to be approached by considering the answer to a series of questions, including:

* Do we *really* know what levels of satisfaction and dissatisfaction exist amongst our patients currently?

* Where patients are dissatisfied, do we *really* know how deep and/or justified this dissatisfaction is?

* Are we *really* aware of the causes of patient irritation with the practice and are there any common strands between any causes for complaint/dissatisfaction that patients might have?

* Do we *really* understand what leads to high(er) levels of patient satisfaction?

* Would we *really* be willing to make possible radical changes in how we operate in order to achieve higher levels of patient satisfaction?

* Have we *really* done enough to train our staff or do we rely upon common-sense and learning from the long-established members of the practice?

* How much money would we *really* be willing to invest in training and facilities in order to achieve higher levels of patient satisfaction?

Given your answers to the questions posed in this chapter and the score from the checklist in Figure 3.3, you should have some understanding of the nature of the practice's orientation and the extent to which it is really patient-centred. Our experience has shown that practices can be viewed very broadly in terms of a continuum, ranging from the inward looking, old-fashioned practice in which patients know their place and dare not move from this, through to the highly patient-centred practice at the other; this is illustrated in Figure 3.4.

The doctor-centred practice is characterized by a belief that:

- general practice has not really changed since the 1930s and change is something that should be resisted

- patients are fundamentally a nuisance

- surgery hours should be based on what is most convenient to the partners

- the practice manager and reception staff are there to keep patients away from the doctors as much as possible

- the surgery building is regarded as a cost, which must be kept to a minimum, rather than an investment

- doctors always know best

The patient-centred practice is characterized by:

- a clear understanding of how the patients' full range of needs might best be satisfied and the benefits they are seeking

- a willingness to adapt the practice and its operating approaches to meet these needs fully

- an understanding of how rival practices operate and what can be learned from them

- a willingness to experiment

- a listening approach

- the development of new and patient-relevant services

- an appointments system which is designed to suit patients' needs

- a willingness to invest in better facilities, including the waiting room

- a well thought out programme of training for medical and non-medical staff

Figure 3.4 The doctor-centred/patient-centred practice continuum

In most cases, of course, practices do not appear at one extreme or the other but are at some point along the continuum. In identifying where on this you are, you should focus less upon the specifics of the factors that characterize doctor-centred and patient-centred practices, but instead upon the nature of the underlying picture and the extent to which this reflects the prevailing attitudes, cultures and methods of operating within your own practice. Having done this and identified which end of the spectrum the practice is biased towards, consider why the practice is where it is. You may well find that the nature of the practice mirrors the general approach of the one or two longest serving and most senior of the partners.

SUMMARY

This chapter has concentrated on some of the dimensions of a patient-centred practice, describing how such an approach can only be developed against the background of a clear and detailed understanding of patients' expectations. In developing a stronger patient orientation, an obvious starting point is the recognition of the distinction between features and benefits and of the need to look outside the practice and evaluate its offer from the patients' perspective. In the absence of this, the practice will almost inevitably lack the patient focus that increasingly is being demanded and expected.

4

Patient satisfaction and the role of marketing research

> Having read this chapter, you should:
>
> - understand the nature and purpose of marketing research;
> - appreciate how it might contribute to the management of the practice;
> - understand how marketing research can be used to measure levels of patient satisfaction;
> - be aware of the factors that need to be taken into account in designing a survey of patients;
> - be capable of designing a straightforward and usable questionnaire.

When the history of the twentieth century comes to be written, the one thing that is certain is that the 1980s and 90s will be labelled decades of change. People today are generally more knowledgeable (something which to a harried receptionist on a busy Monday morning may not always necessarily be particularly obvious) and far more willing to complain (often painfully obvious) than was typically the case in the past. Partly because of changes such as these, but also because the FHSA now has the task of carrying out surveys on patient satisfaction and because patients are much more willing to vote with their feet by moving to another practice if they feel dissatisfied, the need to measure levels of patient satisfaction – and act upon the results – is now greater than ever before. However, in doing this you should not focus just upon the question of how patients interact with the practice, but instead you should take a broader approach so that account is taken of how your patients interact with providers, such as hospitals and individual consultants, when you refer them on for more specialized treatment.

GETTING PATIENT FEEDBACK

Although the idea of getting feedback from patients may well seem attractive since it should provide an insight to what the practice is doing right, what it is doing wrong and what changes might be needed, several questions need to be considered before setting out to conduct any sort of patient survey. These include:

1. Why are you really bothering to measure satisfaction levels?

2. Whose views will you canvass?

3. How frequently will it be done? Will it, for example, be a one-off exercise or something which is done on a regular basis?

4. Who will analyse the results?

5. Who will see the results?

6. How will the results be used?

Although the answers to some of these questions might appear at first sight to be glaringly obvious they are asked in all seriousness. In our work with a number of practices, we have come across several in which surveys of patients have been conducted because they appeared to be a good idea but without any real thought given as to how the results might be used. In other practices we have found that surveys have been conducted and suggestions made, only for one or more of the partners to dismiss the results as meaningless or to argue that the cost of making any of the changes called for is too high.

There are several possible lessons to be learned here. The first is that there must be agreement between the partners, the practice manager and the staff that a survey will be carried out and that the results – good, bad or indifferent – will not only be taken seriously, but will also be used as a basis for future action. Without this there is no point in going any further. It also needs to be agreed that the results will be aggregated to ensure confidentiality and used positively rather than negatively. In one case we came across, for example, a patient made a critical comment about one of the reception staff which ultimately found its way in to the person's annual appraisal. The result was that when the idea of a survey update emerged several months later, the level of support from a large number of the staff was, quite understandably, virtually non-existent.

Even if such an experience might seem unusual and possibly far-fetched, the example has a serious purpose and highlights the fact that survey results can, on occasion, be uncomfortable and that if surveys of patients are to be conducted, they need to be done properly and the results used intelligently and sensitively.

APPROACHES TO RESEARCH

In deciding how to collect patients' views, you have a choice between a series of formal and informal methods. The informal, which include occasional talks with patients, anecdotes and gossip, have little if any real value, since almost invariably they lack the objectivity that you are looking for and indeed require. Undoubtedly, however, in some practices it is these sorts of techniques which predominate and which then provide the basis for subsequent decisions.

The alternative to this is a series of more formal methods which offer far greater potential for gaining an objective and detailed insight to patients' views. The best known of these formal methods are small discussion groups (sometimes called focus groups), evaluation cards and questionnaire-based patient surveys; suggestion boxes, however good and cheap they might appear as a way of getting feedback from patients, rarely prove to be worthwhile.

THE ROLE OF DISCUSSION GROUPS

Discussion groups are now a well-established part of any market researcher's tool kit and involve a group of eight or so people sitting around a table to discuss a particular issue in depth, such as their expectations of the doctor-patient relationship and how their current experiences match these expectations. These groups are of potential value and can generate a considerably detailed insight but they are time consuming (a single group might conceivably last for between one and two hours). They often involve a substantial amount of effort in order to ensure that representative groups appear on time, and require a quiet and undisturbed room as well as a skilled interviewer who is sensitive to the dynamics of the group. On top of all this, it is normal for a token payment (say £20 or a bottle of wine) to be made to the participants.

Partly because of the ways in which the costs of running discussion groups can quickly add up, but also because of the specialized and expensive skills needed to run a discussion group effectively, many practices see evaluation cards and periodic questionnaire-based surveys to be far more flexible and cost-effective methods of obtaining feedback from patients.

EVALUATION CARDS

The thinking behind evaluation cards, an example of which appears in Box 4.1, is straightforward and based on the idea that by asking patients to answer, say, five or six simple questions on the way out of the surgery after the consultation, the practice can monitor standards and perceptions on a low-cost and ongoing basis.

Box 4.1:   A sample evaluation card

As a practice we are committed to improving the service and facilities that we offer to our patients. To help with this, we should be grateful if you would spend a few minutes answering the questions below.

ALL RESULTS ARE TREATED IN ABSOLUTE CONFIDENCE.

1.   Did you have any problems in making a convenient appointment?   Yes/No

2.   Were the reception staff helpful?   Yes/No

3.   How long did you have to wait before seeing the doctor?   . . . mins

4.   Do you feel that the doctor spent enough time with you?   Yes/No

5.   Do you fully understand the doctor's diagnosis and instructions?   Yes/No

6.   How could we improve our service:

Thank you for spending time completing this questionnaire.

DESIGNING A SURVEY

As an alternative to evaluation cards, which by their very nature can give you only a limited amount of information, periodic and more detailed surveys of patients offer considerably greater scope for monitoring attitudes to and perceptions of a far wider range of features within the practice. They also highlight the impact of any changes and any progress that is being made (an example of a questionnaire appears towards the end of the chapter in Box 4.3).

However, before rushing away to begin the work of designing a questionnaire-based survey, several factors need to be borne in mind, including:

- completing all but the very briefest of questionnaires takes time;

- patients may well feel stressed;

- the point at which the questionnaire is answered (eg before or after the consultation) is likely to influence the pattern of answers;

- patients may give you the answers that they think you want.

Other rather more practical issues which need to be taken into account include the need for a table, chair and pen at which self-completion questionnaires can be answered or, if the questions are being asked and the answers recorded by an interviewer, an area in which the patient's answers and comments will not be overheard. One other point that needs to be considered is that some patients are seemingly reluctant to make critical comments, since they believe that if they do this they are likely to be crossed off the doctors' list. Guarantees of the anonymity and confidentiality of the results seem to have little effect in these circumstances.

Nevertheless, despite these minor obstacles and difficulties, surveys, if conducted properly, can be of enormous value, particularly if a series of basic guidelines, which might appear obvious but which all too easily get forgotten in the excitement, are adhered to; these are outlined in Box 4.2.

WHO SHOULD THE SURVEY COVER?

To a very large extent the survey's objectives dictate who precisely should be covered by the survey. In some cases, the nature of the sample is self evident.

Box 4.2:   The guidelines for designing effective questionnaires

- Keep questions short.

- Make sure that the questions are simple and unambiguous.

- Don't ask questions which lead respondents to a particular answer.

- Try not to ask too many questions (10 is a reasonable number, 12 or 13 is probably the absolute maximum in these circumstances).

- Allow respondents to be anonymous.

- Avoid potentially embarrassing questions.

- Wherever possible, use questions which allow respondents either to give simple 'Yes/No' answers or use a rating scale, since they make the job of analysis far easier. Open ended questions (eg 'Do you have any suggestions for how the range of services might be improved?') can give interesting answers but often take a great deal of time to analyse.

- Work out in advance how the results will be analysed and used (a good tip is that students from a local college, particularly if they are on a Business Studies course, may well be able to help in the development of a question-naire, as well as in the analysis of the results and preparation of the report).

- Include a section at the end of the questionnaire which will allow you to classify respondents by age, sex, marital status, or any other dimension (eg frequency of visits to the surgery) which is considered to be significant.

- Having designed the questionnaire, 'pilot' it on a small number of patients to check that any ambiguities and other problems can be ironed out.

If, for example, you are interested in the reactions of mothers of newly-born children to their ante-natal care, the question of who to approach is not difficult. For a study with a rather broader purpose, such as identifying general levels of satisfaction with appointment times, reception areas, and so on, a representative cross section of patients will be needed.

With regard to the numbers of people who will be covered by the study, a key constraint is often that of the amount of time and effort involved in the analysis. On the face of it, although the administration and analysis of 200 completed questionnaires may seem manageable, remember that if each questionnaire consists of just ten questions, this generates 2,000 answers that will need to be looked at and analysed, all of which will probably have to be done by the practice manager on top of his or her normal day-to-day pressures. Because of this, a rather more pragmatic approach would involve dealing with, say, 30 or 40 questionnaires a week for four or five weeks or, as suggested earlier, asking a student to do the work for you.

Box 4.3:   An example of a patient satisfaction questionnaire

As a practice, we are committed to improving the range of facilities and the quality of the service that we offer to our patients. To help us with this, we should be grateful if you would spend a few minutes completing this questionnaire.

ALL RESULTS WILL BE TREATED IN ABSOLUTE CONFIDENCE.

Please give a rating to each of the following elements of the practice by putting a tick in the appropriate box.

	Good	Adequate	Bad
1. The appointment system and:			
(a) getting through by telephone to make an appointment	❑	❑	❑
(b) being able to make an appointment at a time that is convenient	❑	❑	❑
(c) the doctor or nurse's punctuality	❑	❑	❑
2. The receptionists and their:			
(a) helpfulness	❑	❑	❑
(b) friendliness	❑	❑	❑
(c) efficiency	❑	❑	❑
3. The waiting room and its:			
(a) level of comfort	❑	❑	❑
(b) range of facilities	❑	❑	❑
(c) cleanliness	❑	❑	❑
(d) tidiness	❑	❑	❑
4. The consultation with the doctor or nurse and:			
(a) the amount of time spent with you	❑	❑	❑
(b) the doctor or nurse's friendliness	❑	❑	❑
(c) the doctor or nurse's helpfulness	❑	❑	❑

continued over

Box 4.3: *continued*

	Yes	No
5. Having seen the doctor or nurse, do you fully understand the diagnosis and instructions?	❏	❏
6. Are you fully aware of the procedures for obtaining repeat prescriptions?	❏	❏

7. Are you aware of the following services that we offer?

	Yes	No
Well man/well woman	❏	❏
Family planning	❏	❏
Immunization/vaccination	❏	❏
Ante-natal	❏	❏
Relaxation	❏	❏
Diabetic advice	❏	❏
Stress/hypertension	❏	❏
Dieting	❏	❏
Stop smoking	❏	❏
Bereavement counselling	❏	❏

8. Has the doctor ever referred you to the hospital for an appointment for tests or further examination?

Yes ❏   If yes, please go to question 9

No ❏   If no, please go to question 10

9. How would your rate the hospital staff and their:

	Good	Adequate	Bad
(a) helpfulness	❏	❏	❏
(b) friendliness	❏	❏	❏
(c) efficiency	❏	❏	❏

and the hospital consultants:

	Good	Adequate	Bad
(a) willingness to listen	❏	❏	❏
(b) willingness to explain	❏	❏	❏
(c) helpfulness	❏	❏	❏

continued opposite

Box 4.3:   *continued*

	Good	Adequate	Bad
10. Taking all of these factors into account, how would you rate the overall quality of the services that you have received from us?	❑	❑	❑

11. Do you have any suggestions of how we might improve the service we offer to you?

12. Now please give us a few details about yourself

Sex:	male	❑	female	❑
Age:	18–29	❑		
	30–39	❑		
	40–49	❑		
	50–64	❑		
	65+	❑		

13. How frequently do you *normally* attend surgery? (please tick)

Once a week	❑
Once a month	❑
Once or twice a year	❑
Three to four times a year	❑
Less frequently than once a year	❑

Thank you for spending the time to complete this questionnaire.

AFTER THE SURVEY

Having completed the survey, you then have to face the question of how the results will be presented to the staff. Insofar as it is possible to give advice on this, you should be as open as possible. Your staff will be only too aware that a survey of patients has been conducted and want to know what has been said. Given this, you should aim to produce a summary of key findings – positive as well as negative – within a week or so of the survey being finished and circulate this to everyone in the practice, together with an outline of exactly how the results will be used in the future management of the practice.

SUMMARY

Within this chapter we have focused upon some of the ways in which you might obtain feedback from patients and measure the levels of satisfaction that exist. In this context, you might usefully consider the following questions:

1. If you were to go ahead with a survey of patients, who would have the responsibility for managing the survey by developing the questionnaire, analysing the results and preparing the report?

2. What information do you feel you really need to manage the practice more effectively?

3. What do you feel would be the best ways in which to collect this information?

4. How will you present the results to the staff?

5

Environmental pressures and the parable of the boiled frog

Having read this chapter, you should:

- understand the various dimensions of the macro and micro external environments and how their patterns of interaction are capable of affecting the practice;

- understand the need to review the environment on a regular basis;

- appreciate how the environment creates opportunities and threats;

- have an insight to the ways in which the practice environment is likely to develop and become more volatile over the next few years;

- understand the implications of this for approaches to practice organization.

We commented in Chapter two that marketing involves a four-stage process: environmental analysis; planning; implementation; and feedback and control. Here we focus upon the first of these and examine the significance of the practice's environment, the ways in which it is changing, the implications of this and how an understanding of the probable patterns of environmental change is capable of contributing to more effective marketing planning. However, before looking at the detail of this, it is worth learning the lesson of the boiled frog.

THE PARABLE OF THE BOILED FROG

All organizations are faced with a series of environmental changes and challenges. The principle difference between the effective and the ineffective organization is how well it responds, something that was encapsulated several years ago in one of the most popular of management fables, the parable of the boiled frog. What is now referred to as 'the boiled frog syndrome' is based on the idea that if you drop a frog into a pan of very hot water, it instantly leaps out. If, however, you put a frog into a pan of lukewarm water and turn the heat up very slowly, it sits there quite happily not noticing the change in its environment. The frog, of course, eventually dies.

The parallels with the management and development of the practice are, or should be, apparent. Faced with sudden and dramatic environmental change, the need for a response is obvious. Faced with a much slower pace of change, the pressures to respond are far less (ie the 'we are doing reasonably well and can reassess things at some time in the future' phenomenon), with the result that the organization becomes increasingly distant from the real demands of its customers (patients) and other stakeholders. Given this, think hard about whether you are one of the frogs that is sitting quite happily in a pan of increasingly hot water. If so, why, what are the possible consequences and what, if anything, are you going to do about it?

ANALYSING THE PRACTICE ENVIRONMENT

Although a variety of frameworks have been developed to help the process of analysing the environment and assessing its probable effect upon an organization, the most useful of these is referred to as PEST analysis, with PEST representing an acronym of what are the four major dimensions of the environment for the majority of organizations: the Political/legal; Economic/competitive; Socio-cultural; and Technological elements.

The thinking that underpins PEST analysis is straightforward and involves taking each of the four elements in turn, identifying the nature and significance of any changes that are likely to take place both in the short-term and long-term, and then assessing what effect these will have upon the organization. Having done this, thought can then be given to the actions and responses that are possible and/or demanded.

Although the relative importance of the four factors may vary over time, and indeed their impact may be either direct or indirect, the benefits of regular environmental analysis can be considerable. They are reflected most obviously by a practice that is capable of behaving far more proactively, recognizing opportunities and threats at an earlier stage and taking the action that is needed in order to capitalize on the opportunities and minimize or avoid altogether the impact of any threats.

It follows that if you are to act in a proactive manner, you need to begin by identifying and categorizing those parts of the environment over which you are able to exert at least some small degree of control, and those which, by virtue of being totally outside your control, need to be seen as environmental constraints. Having done this you can then start to develop a strategy which is far more likely to reflect environment pressures and realities rather than the partners' preconceived and possibly misconceived, ideas of what is feasible.

The reality for many small organizations, and we include general practice within this, is that the vast majority of external factors are constraints which only rarely can be changed or influenced to any real degree. The implications of this are, firstly, that the argument for monitoring the environment is inescapable since you need to shape the practice so that it more accurately reflects environmental demands, and secondly, that you need to structure the practice so that it is sufficiently flexible to be able to respond effectively and quickly to external pressures, be they in the form of opportunities or threats.

THE STRUCTURE OF THE ENVIRONMENT

The various dimensions of the environment are illustrated in Figure 5.1. It can be seen from this that the environment in capable of being categorized not just on the basis of the PEST factors, but also on the basis of their macro nature, in that they effect the nation as a whole (an obvious example would be the changing demographic patterns and in particular the increasing numbers of elderly people) as well as their micro impact, in that they have a direct and immediate effect upon the practice or the local area. An example of this would be the way in which an upsurge in local levels of unemployment generally has a knock on effect upon patterns of health in the communities involved.

Because of the ways in which the environment is the immediate or ultimate influence upon patterns of demand for the practice's services, a regular environmental review is capable of providing significant information not just on the sort of changes taking place but also on the patterns of response and development within the practice that are called for. Without this, it is likely that sooner or later the practice will be forced into a series of reactive responses in a desperate attempt to avoid the sort of mismatch between the demands of

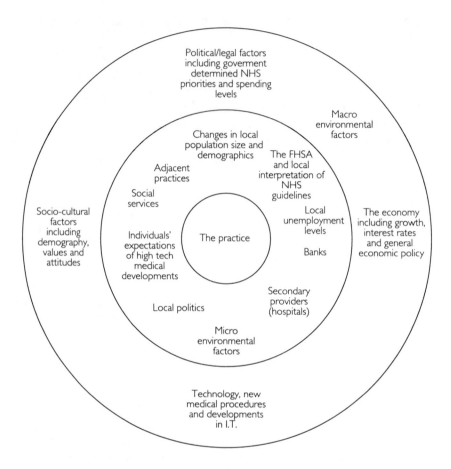

Figure 5.1:   The practice environment

the environment and what the practice is actually offering; this mismatch is illustrated in Figure 5.2.

The phenomenon that Figure 5.2 illustrates is sometimes referred to as 'strategic drift' and is one that we have encountered in a great many practices and is manifested in a variety of ways. Among these is a failure on the part of the partners to recognize and agree how emerging opportunities might be exploited, growing levels of patient dissatisfaction, little desire amongst the staff to carry out anything other than routine tasks, and a general weakening in the image of the practice both within the community and the health service. Faced with this, the only response that is left is a radical reassessment of what the

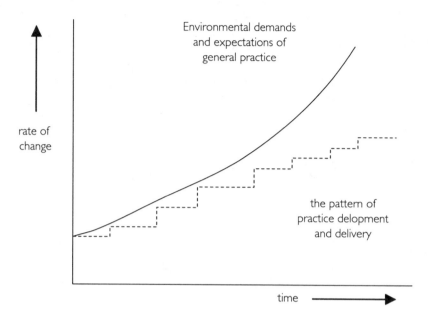

Figure 5.2: The mismatch between the environmental demands and practice delivery

environment is demanding of the practice currently, how this is likely to change and how the practice intends responding in order to catch up.

PATTERNS OF ENVIRONMENTAL CHANGES

In looking at any environment, we can categorize it on the basis of the nature and pace of the changes taking place, and the organizational implications of this. In Figure 5.3 we illustrate four broad patterns of environment change: stability; gradual and largely predictable change; a state of flux; and chaos.

In general practice, the sort of environmental changes faced by GPs for a long time correspond to stage two, that of gradual and largely predictable patterns which could be managed with few real problems. Over the past few years, however, it is not only the pace and scale of change that has increased dramatically, but also the degree of unpredictability. Thus the nature and speed of the responses that are required have escalated enormously. In organizational terms, the relevance of this can be examined under a number of headings, but particularly in terms of the need for greater practice flexibility, better patterns of communication and higher levels of staff training.

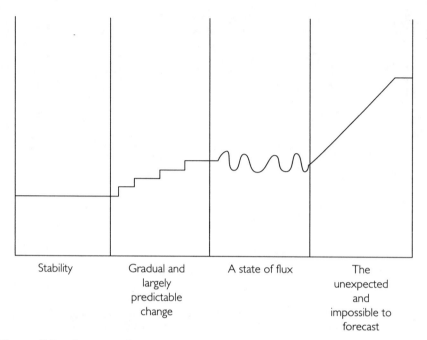

| Stability | Gradual and largely predictable change | A state of flux | The unexpected and impossible to forecast |

Figure 5.3: Patterns of environmental change

THE SIGNIFICANCE OF SOCIAL CHANGE

Perhaps the most significant series of changes that general practice will have to be reconciled with over the next few years stems from the series of structural and altitudinal shifts that are taking place within society. Included within these are:

- the growing number of elderly people and a series of other major demographic shifts;
- the gap that is widening between the haves and the have-nots;
- a growth in the number of single parents;
- a decline in the nuclear family as divorce rates rise;
- changes in family structures;
- lifestyle changes;
- changes in smoking and drinking patterns;

- different attitudes to health and fitness;

- changing attitudes to institutional responses and a desire for more personal and individual treatment;

- a greater willingness to complain and resort to remedial action;

- expectations of higher service levels.

Although this is not a comprehensive list, it provides an indication of the sorts of social changes that are likely to have an impact over the next few years. Recognizing this, you should go through the list, adding to it where necessary, and assess the extent to which you feel that your practice will be affected by each of the points and, then how you might respond most effectively.

Together, however, they spell out the need for more flexible and organic approaches to practice organization. The alternative, a largely traditional and mechanistic structure, simply creates problems. Consider therefore, the questions that appear in Box 5.1.

Box 5.1:   How effectively has your practice responded to and managed change?

1.   What are the biggest changes that you feel have affected general practice over the last few years?
2.   Which of the changes that have taken place have had the greatest effect upon:
     (a)   your practice; and
     (b)   you as a member of the practice?
3.   Overall, how well do you think that these changes have been handled?
4.   What have been the major problems that have been experienced in responding to and managing these changes?
5.   What are the principal causes of these problems?
6.   What, if anything, has been done and is being done to overcome these problems?
7.   What do you see to be the major changes that the practice will have to face up to over the next few years?
8.   How well equipped is the practice to deal with these effectively?
9.   What areas of managerial strength and weakness exist in the practice?
10. What messages do they send out about your ability to handle future change effectively?

In answering these, you need to give serious thought not just to the superficial changes that have been initiated in the practice, but rather to the more fundamental issues of the attitude and behaviour of everyone (partners and staff) in the practice. We know of some practices, for example, which have installed impressive computer systems, changed the titles of some of the staff and even moved to new premises, but which still think and act in the same way that they have for years with no real improvement in their organization, style of leadership or approaches to teamworking. They are now suffering the problems of substantially worse staff morale which has lead us to identify four different types of practice; these are illustrated in Box 5.2.

Although there is an obvious element of parody in at least two of these profiles, there is a more important, underlying question which is concerned with the attitudes to change that exist within the practice, how well the practice has responded to change so far, the extent to which planning for the future is going on, and the quality of this planning. The question of how well the practice has responded so far was considered in Box 5.1 and may well have highlighted whether your responses to change have been planned or were largely fortuitous. In dealing with the quality of planning for the future, you need to give thought to two interrelated issues: firstly, the extent to which there is a fundamental recognition on the part of the doctors and staff of the need to continue changing over the next few years and secondly, the willingness to make these changes proactively rather than simply responding to them. This is illustrated in Figure 5.4 on page 52.

Having placed the practice within this matrix, ask yourself a few straightforward questions:

- Why are we in this cell of the matrix?

- Are we happy with this? If so, what do we have to do either to stay here or improve yet further?

- If we are not happy with the current position, what are the root causes and what do we have to do to improve things?

Box 5.2:   The four types of practice and their responses to change

The dinosaurs

Practices which exist in a time warp. Life goes on as it always has, with few if any changes. In essence, it is the sort of practice which, when you are sitting in the waiting room, you have the chance to read the article in the Reader's Digest or National Geographic which you missed on its first time round in 1953. The floors are covered with linoleum, the walls are painted a shade of hospital green that is guaranteed to induce a degree of nausea in even the healthiest of patients, the reception staff see the surgery as their personal fiefdom, patients are an unwelcome intrusion and friendliness is seen as a sign of weakness, whilst the doctors regret the changes that have led to leeches no longer being a central part of any treatment. The patient list is small and declining and made up of primarily elderly patients who have been on the list for years and who would find the transfer to another practice impossible even to contemplate. Change is seen as a nuisance, a threat and largely unnecessary, with the result that the partners work hard to avoid any move away from the methods of operation which were at the cutting edge of practice management in the 1920s.

The docile and contented cows that are ambling along

Practices that have made steady if unspectacular incremental progress. The waiting room has been spruced up, the magazines are circa 1981, the staff have name badges, a computer has been installed, the inputting of data has begun and the partners regularly attend PGEA events in order to find out about the latest medical and management advances. The partners are waiting to discover the outcome of the next general election before deciding whether to become fundholders. The decision should coincide with the first real outputs from the computer.

The sheep

The sort of practice in which the senior partner has latched on to and introduced every new idea that has come along in the last five years only to replace it after a couple of months with something new. There is little evidence of planning or of a well thought out and sustained direction, but considerable evidence of a series of knee-jerk responses to a variety of half-baked ideas. The computer system is impressive.

The eagles

Practices in which considerable thought has been given to the future and to the sorts of objectives that are most appropriate. These thoughts have then been reflected in a series of considered and appropriate responses that take full account of the various stakeholders' expectations. The result is a practice that is well prepared to cope with the challenges of the next few years, but in which complacency, partner rivalry, obstruction and self-satisfaction has no place.

Recognition on the part of the
doctors and staff of the need for
further and possibly radical
change

Low   High

	Low	High
Low	Ostriches burying their heads in the sand	Rabbits mesmerized by the approaching headlights
High	Lizards basking in the sun but seeing no need to change currently	Road runners which are constantly alert and know which direction to go

The willingness to
make these
changes

Figure 5.4:   The change matrix

THE STEPS IN ANALYSING THE ENVIRONMENT

Box 5.3 provides a broad framework that is designed to help in the process of identifying how the environment is likely to change over the next few years, what the implications for the practice will probably be, and what the strategic imperatives are (a strategic imperative is a 'must do' factor; unaddressed, the consequences for the practice are likely to be significant). Having done this, you can then move on to Boxes 5.4–5.7 which require you to look more specifically at the four individual dimensions of the environment that we referred to earlier, identify the specific changes taking place, assess whether these represent opportunities or threats, and what action the practice needs to take.

To do this, you should work your way through each of these areas with your partners with a view to identifying, firstly, the nature of any changes that are likely to take place and subsequently, what this entails for the practice. Use a flipchart and brainstorm so that as many ideas as possible are generated without

Box 5.3:   Basic environmental beliefs, their implications and the strategic imperatives that emerge from this

Basic environmental beliefs

I believe that the following environmental changes will take place over the next few years:	The implications for the practice of each of these changes will be:	The strategic imperatives (the must-dos) that emerge are:
1.	1.	1.
2.	2.	2.
3.	3.	3.
4.	4.	4.
5.	5.	5.
6.	6.	6.
7.	7.	7.
8.	8.	8.
9.	9.	9.
10.	10.	10.

being evaluated or criticized. Once you have done this, go back and assess each of the ideas before entering them into the Boxes.

The political/legal framework

- What sorts of changes in the present government's policies do you foresee?

- What might a change in the government mean for the NHS in general and spending patterns in particular?

- What changes do you foresee in FHSA priorities?

- What effects would a change in funding levels for local social services have?

- What changes do you foresee in the levels of doctors' responsibility and accountability?

- What changes seem likely in the incentives given to members of the public to take private health insurance?

- Who within the practice has the responsibility for keeping the partners up to date on the relevant medico-legal changes?

Box 5.4:   Probable PEST developments

The political environment

The probable developments are . . .	The probable, specific effects upon the practice are . . .	Do these represent an opportunity or a threat?	What do we need to do to capitalize upon the opportunity or minimize the threat?
•	• • •	• • •	• • •
•	• • •	• • •	• • •
•	• • •	• • •	• • •
•	• • •	• • •	• • •

The economic, competitive and provider environments

- What changes do you expect to see in economic conditions?

- How will unemployment levels move locally and what are the implications for patterns of health?

- In what ways is competition becoming more significant for general practice and how is this affecting you?

- What changes are likely to take place amongst other suppliers of medical services, such as osteopaths and chiropodists, and what are the implications for general practice?

- What sort of relationship do you have with your neighbouring practices?

- What appear to be their objectives and how are they likely to develop over the next few years? Do their patterns of development have any implications for you?

- What might you learn from how other practices operate?

- Is there any scope for co-operation?

Box 5.5:   Probable PEST developments

The economic/competitive environment

The probable developments are . . .	The probable, specific effects upon the practice are . . .	Do these represent an opportunity or a threat?	What do we need to do to capitalize upon the opportunity or minimize the threat?
•	• • •	• • •	• • •
•	• • •	• • •	• • •
•	• • •	• • •	• • •
•	• • •	• • •	• • •

- What changes do you expect to see in relationships with providers, such as hospitals and individual consultants?

The social and cultural environments

- What social changes do you expect to see over the next few years?
- What are the implications for you of trends and shifts in the local population size and demographic structures?
- In what ways are patients' expectations of general practice changing?
- In what ways are values and lifestyles changing?
- What new social and cultural pressures and priorities are emerging?

Box 5.6:   Probable PEST developments

The socio-cultural environment

The probable developments are . . .	The probable, specific effects upon the practice are . . .	Do these represent an opportunity or a threat?	What do we need to do to capitalize upon the opportunity or minimize the threat?
•	• • •	• • •	• • •
•	• • •	• • •	• • •
•	• • •	• • •	• • •
•	• • •	• • •	• • •

The technological environment

- How will technological changes and developments affect general practice over the next few years?

- In what ways are individuals' expectations of higher technology clinical solutions likely to develop?

- What are the implications for your spending patterns of new technological developments?

- Are you and your partners fully up to date with the nature and patterns of technological developments in medicine?

- How can you use new technology to improve your range and level of services?

- Does anyone within the practice have the specific responsibility for monitoring new developments and keeping the others informed?

Box 5.7:   Probable PEST developments

The technological environment

The probable developments are . . .	The probable, specific effects upon the practice are . . .	Do these represent an opportunity or a threat?	What do we need to do to capitalize upon the opportunity or minimize the threat?
•	• • •	• • •	• • •
•	• • •	• • •	• • •
•	• • •	• • •	• • •
•	• • •	• • •	• • •

Once this exercise is complete you should have a far clearer and more focused view of how the practice environment is likely to develop and what the implications of this are likely to be. Armed with this information, you can begin identifying in detail the sorts of opportunities and threats that exist, the ways in which they are most likely to develop in the near future and how they can best be handled; a framework for this appears in Box 5.8.

Box 5.8:   The opportunities and threats facing the practice

The opportunities open to us appear to be . . .	Their significance (1–5) (1 = of little significance) (5 = of major significance)	The actions that are needed to capitalize upon the opportunities are . . .
• • • •		• • • •
The threats facing us appear to be . . .	Their significance (1–5)	The actions needed to minimize the possible impact of the threats are . . .
• • • • •		• • • •

SUMMARY

Within this chapter, we have focused upon the various dimensions of the environment and described how an understanding of the environment and the ways in which it is likely to change underpins any worthwhile approach to planning. In the light of this, consider the following questions:

1. Do you feel that you have a sufficiently detailed understanding of how the practice environment is likely to change over the next few years?

2. What sort of environment does it look as if you will have to face up to?

3. How confident are you that you will be able to cope effectively?

4. Where do the greatest opportunities and threats appear to be?

5. Given your previous patterns of behaviour, how are you most likely to respond to any changes? Will it be very largely in the form of a series of almost desperate moves or in a much more systematic and planned manner?

Finally, return for a moment to the story of the boiled frog and think not just about the lessons that arise from this but also, considering your responses to the questions that we have raised within this chapter, what sort of frog you *really* are.

6

Planning for success (part one): assessing your planning skills

> Having read this chapter, you should:
>
> • understand more clearly what you want from planning;
> • have a greater understanding of the planning skills and abilities possessed by you and your colleagues.

SO WHAT DO YOU WANT FROM PLANNING?

It has long been recognized that planning is generally a relatively easy and straightforward exercise and that the development of a truly worthwhile plan takes only a little more time and effort than that involved in preparing one which is mediocre. The problems that many organizations face come not at the planning stage but are instead related to the ways in which the plan is implemented. Far too often, for example, too few resources are put into the process of implementation and responsibilities are only loosely allocated, with the result that objectives are not achieved within the intended timescales. Faced with this, the all too common reaction, particularly when the environment is changing rapidly, is that planning is of little real value and the process becomes no more than a hollow exercise.

If, however, the processes of planning and implementation are seen to be interconnected, responsibilities are properly allocated, and someone within the practice takes on the task of 'driving' the plan, the benefits can be considerable and reflected in a far tighter focus and much higher levels of motivation and performance.

Yet, for many managers, and we include GPs within this, planning runs the risk of taking on what is sometimes loosely referred to as 'motherhood' status.

In other words, it is warm, reassuring and difficult to argue against. Before we go any further, therefore, you need to consider seven simple questions:

1. Why are you bothering to plan?

2. What will the plan be used for?

3. How will it be used?

4. Who will be involved in the planning process?

5. Who will write it (and how)?

6. Who will manage and drive it?

7. What measures of success will you use?

In working with a wide variety of organizations over the years, it has become apparent that when it comes to planning, there are two broad approaches. The first is characterized by an emphasis upon producing a lengthy, detailed, highly polished and professional-looking plan which either literally or figuratively is filed until the start of the next year's planning cycle.

The second approach, and the one which we want to give emphasis in this chapter, gives full recognition to the benefits of the planning *process*; it provides a forum for a detailed review of the environment, objectives, priorities, resources, strengths and weaknesses, and the alternative patterns of proactive development that exist. This is then reflected in the plan itself which represents a *working document* which is used on a daily or weekly basis to manage the practice.

Given this, the answer to the first of the seven questions posed above has to be that any plan that is developed must be realistic and designed to make a major contribution to the management of the practice, rather than to satisfy any guidelines or expectations of bodies such as the FHSA. It follows from this that you need to think about developing a *planning culture* within the practice in which the process of planning is taken seriously rather than as a once-a-year ritual.

BEING REALISTIC ABOUT YOUR PLANNING SKILLS

Perhaps one of the most common complaints that we have heard from doctors over the past two years is that they became doctors to practice medicine rather than to become professional managers. Although we have a certain sympathy for this view, few GPs today are able to duck their management and planning responsibilities. However, recognizing that doctors vary enormously in terms of their planning abilities, a first stage in developing an effective planning process involves being realistic (perhaps brutally honest would be a better phrase) about the planning skills of each of the partners within the practice.

To do this, begin with the matrix that appears in Figure 6.1 which requires you to categorize individuals on the basis of two dimensions: their apparent long-term planning abilities and their skills in day-to-day management. Using this matrix, identify where you, your partners and the practice manager are located. The picture that emerges from this should give you a reasonable insight to the overall quality of management and the planning strengths that exist within the practice, whether there is a need to strengthen these, and who might be best equipped to take on the initial responsibility for planning (this is not necessarily the senior partner). In completing this matrix, you are also arriving at a measure of what is loosely referred to as organizational capability; that is the practice's capacity for handling change and moving ahead in the right direction.

	Their long-term planning abllities	
	Low	High
Low Their effectiveness as a day-to-day manager	The bumblers and the dodos who are out of touch and who are unlikely to survive or grow in the long-term	The long sighted stumblers who constantly experience short-term problems
High	The myopics who will stagnate	The visionaries who will thrive

Figure 6.1:   The short and long-term management skills matrix

Against this background, you should then move to Figure 6.2 which enables you to categorize yourself and your colleagues on the basis of their willingness to manage and their ability to manage; the four types that this produces are discussed in Box 6.1.

Their ability to manage effectively

Their willingness to manage	Low	High
Low	The incompetent meddlers	The opt-outs and ostriches
High	The dangermedics	The supermedics

Figure 6.2: The four GP management styles

Box 6.1: The four types of doctor-manager

In the light of a study that we conducted amongst practice managers in 1993 to find out how they viewed their GPs as managers, we identified four types of doctor-manager: the supermedics; the dangermedics; the opt-outs and ostriches; and the incompetent meddlers.

The **supermedic** proved to be an all too rare and unnerving species but is immediately recognizable by an evangelical gleam in his or her eye, an almost pathological commitment to change, a passion for computerization, and a love of plans, planning and staff information notes. Supermedics tend to put enormous emphasis on mission statements for the practice, partners' away days in order to decide on the future objectives and shape of the practice, staff motivation, and scrupulous record keeping. Their briefcases bulge with business plans and a mobile phone sits next to the stethoscope.

The **dangermedics** are the GPs who, despite few obvious managerial skills, are intent on demonstrating to staff throughout the practice that they are in charge and are full of ideas (few of which are original and fewer still are understood). They tend to use management jargon indiscriminately and are intent on bringing about change; in managerial terms they are the equivalent of someone practising as a doctor having failed their Boy Scouts or Girl Guides first aid badge. All too often, the sorts of changes they make and the systems they introduce are either inappropriate or, because of a lack of planning and commitment, fail to achieve the hoped for results. Despite this, they insist on being involved in everything and often feel that their staff have no real skills or abilities. Because of this, they have an almost neurotic compulsion to give orders to anyone and everyone. Like the supermedics, dangermedics can be recognized in a number of ways, but most obviously by the trail of confusion and/or destruction they leave behind and their

continued over

Box 6.1: *continued*

insistence upon being consulted about every aspect of the practice. Insofar as they have a pet phrase, it is likely to be either 'Didn't I tell you about that? I suppose I must have forgotten,' or 'Why has it gone wrong? Can't anyone around here do anything right?'

The **opt-outs and ostriches** are something of a disappointment, since although they have a well-developed ability to manage, they either do not see themselves as managers, and consequently leave others to do it, or still have not come to terms with the ways in which general practice has changed over the past few years. Tolerant of a degree of chaos, they often develop delegation to a fine art. Insofar as they can be recognized by what they say as opposed to what they do not do, it is likely to be something along the lines of 'I didn't come into medicine to be a manager, I just want to get on with being a doctor.'

The **incompetent meddlers** proved to be surprisingly common and a source of enormous frustration for many practice managers. These are the GPs who consistently fail to complete vital records on time, rarely if ever tell the staff what is going on or where they are going, see no need to plan, frequently change their mind for no apparent reason, insist on being consulted (a bit like dangermedics), and either would not recognize a practice plan if it landed on their desk or would not be able to find it amongst the mess of free gifts from reps, unanswered telephone messages, half-eaten sandwiches, and still-to-be read articles from the medical press.

SUMMARY

Quite deliberately, within this chapter, we have tried to adopt a light-hearted tone in order to drive home an important message. Given the far greater emphasis upon, and indeed the need for planning in the current climate, it is essential that you have a clear understanding of the managerial and planning strengths that exist within the practice. Without this understanding, there is a danger that you will start with the assumption that all partners have an equal ability and that the responsibilities both for planning and implementation can be shared equally. If our experiences with numerous managers in a wide variety of organizational types over the past twenty years are at all typical, this is simply not the case. It is the recognition of this and the pictures that emerge from the various matrices used in this chapter that prompts us to suggest that it is only after you have identified the level and nature of the planning and managerial

skills within the practice, that the question of who is to be responsible for developing and then subsequently implementing the plan can really be decided.
In summary, therefore, consider the following questions:

1. What overall picture emerges from the various matrices?

2. Does it appear that you have sufficient long-term planning skills amongst the partners and practice managers? If not, what are the probable consequences of this and what might you do to overcome the problem?

7

Planning for success (part two): developing the marketing plan

Having read this chapter, you should:

- understand the nature, purpose and benefits of planning;

- have an appreciation of the sorts of problems that are typically encountered in planning;

- understand the structure of the marketing plan and the input that it requires;

- be aware of how the assumptions that underpin the plan subsequently drive the plan;

- appreciate how stakeholders' needs can be taken into account;

- recognize the factors that influence the effectiveness of the plan's implementation.

Against the background of our comments in Chapters five and six and, hopefully, with a better understanding of the planning skills and abilities that exist within the practice, we can now turn our attention to the question of how best to prepare an effective marketing plan.

THE THREE DIMENSIONS OF PLANNING

All too often plans fail because too little attention is paid to issues of implementation. Equally, plans fail because the objectives that have been set are either too ambitious or fail to reflect the realities of the environment and/or the organization's strengths and capabilities. Recognizing this, planning, which is designed to provide the organization with a sense of direction and purpose, must take place with a clear and detailed understanding of three principal factors:

1. The nature and demands of the environment;
2. The objectives and expectations of the doctors and staff;
3. The practice's strengths, weaknesses and overall levels of capability.

THE STRUCTURE OF THE MARKETING PLAN

There is no one model of the ideal marketing plan but it is relatively easy to identify the twelve areas that need to be included within any worthwhile and usable planning document; these are listed in Box 7.1 and then brought together diagramatically in the model of the planning process in Figure 7.1.

DEVELOPING AN EFFECTIVE PLAN

Planning is based on asking – and answering – three principal questions:

1. Where are we currently?
2. Where do we want to go?
3. How are we going to get there?

The significance of the first of these – where are we currently? – has been highlighted by the ex-chairman of ICI and star of BBC television's *Trouble-shooter* series, Sir John Harvey-Jones:

> 'There is no point in deciding where your business is going until you have actually decided with great clarity where you are now. Like practically everything in business, however, this is easier said than done.'

Box 7.1:   The elements of a marketing plan

1. The summary or overview

2. The situational analysis that includes:
    *   the assumptions about environmental pressures and demands and the assessment of the opportunities and threats that exist currently and which seem likely to emerge during the period covered by the plan
    *   the assessment of the practice's strengths and weaknesses, its overall level of capability and the identification of any significant gaps

3. The implications of the analysis of strengths, weaknesses, opportunities and threats

4. The principal assumptions underlying the plan

5. The statement of the mission and the short and long term marketing objectives

6. The statement of the strategy that is to be pursued

7. The detail of the tactical actions needed

8. The allocation of responsibilities and timescales

9. The resource implications of the plan

10. Feedback mechanisms

11. The performance measures that are to be used to assess the ongoing performance

This stage of the planning process is therefore concerned very largely with identifying the practice's real strengths and weaknesses, along with the nature of any opportunities and threats that exist currently or which seem likely to emerge during the period that is to be covered by the plan. Having done this, you can then move on to the question of the direction in which you want to take the practice, something which involves the development, not just of a clear statement of objectives, but also a vision of the sort of practice that you are trying to develop. With this clear, you can then turn your attention to identifying how this vision and the objectives might best be achieved.

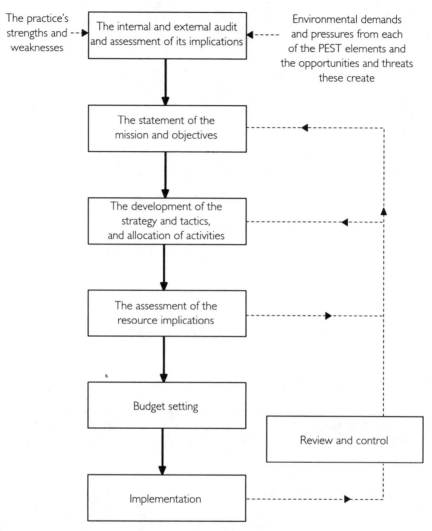

Figure 7.1:   The planning process

STEP ONE

Where are we currently?

How to conduct a SWOT analysis that is really worthwhile
SWOT analysis (Strengths, Weaknesses, Opportunities and Threats) has proved to be one of the most commonly used and abused managerial and planning tools of the past decade.

There are several reasons for this, but perhaps the most obvious is that the technique's apparent simplicity has lulled its users into a false sense of security with the result that time and again the outcome of the analysis is far too bland and meaningless to provide a worthwhile base for planning. Given this, how then can SWOT analysis be made more rigorous and valid? The guidelines developed from experiences with a variety of different types of organization are straightforward.

- Concentrate upon building a picture of the practice as a whole by carrying out a series of preliminary analyses of different parts of the practice. By doing this, you are far less likely to miss some of the detail that needs to come from a SWOT and will gain a much greater insight into how different parts of the practice are operating and need to develop.

- Do not conduct the analysis single-handed, but instead use it as an opportunity for the partners and the staff to pool ideas.

- Always examine strengths and weaknesses through the eyes of the patients and other stakeholders. In this way, you are more likely to avoid making warm, reassuring and motherhood statements about the practice and can concentrate instead upon identifying how the practice is *really* seen from the outside.

- In looking at strengths and weaknesses, start with a broadly unstructured approach in order to get ideas flowing, but gradually pull the points together under a series of headings so that you can build up a picture of the practice's different dimensions. The sorts of headings that you might use in doing this, include:
  - the doctors and other medical staff within the practice;
  - the support and admin staff;
  - skill levels;
  - the premises, including their location;
  - the administrative procedures;
  - the information technology that is being used;
  - financial issues and any investment needed;
  - relationships with patients;
  - relationships with the FHSA;
  - relationships with suppliers, including hospitals;
  - the general reputation of the practice.

- In looking at opportunities and threats in the external environment, concentrate upon those parts of the environment that are likely to have a direct rather than an indirect effect upon the practice.

- Avoid the temptation simply to list strengths, weaknesses, opportunities and threats, since this tends to lead to what we can refer to as a 'balance sheet' mentality; here you take comfort from the way in which, for example, the number of strengths identified outweighs the number of weaknesses. Instead, spend time evaluating each of the points identified and then rank them in order of importance; a framework for doing this appears in Box 7.2.

- Concentrate upon identifying how the results of the analysis can be used. In the case of strengths, for example, there has to be a matching opportunity as without this, the strength is of little, real or immediate value. Equally, in the case of weaknesses, consider how each weakness can be overcome or its significance reduced. In the case of threats, again think of how their impact can be neutralized or reduced, and possibly turned into an opportunity; the framework for this appears in Figure 7.2.

Box 7.2:   Identifying and ranking the practice's strengths, weaknesses, opportunities and threats

Strengths	Significance
Weaknesses	Significance
Opportunities	Significance
Threats	Significance

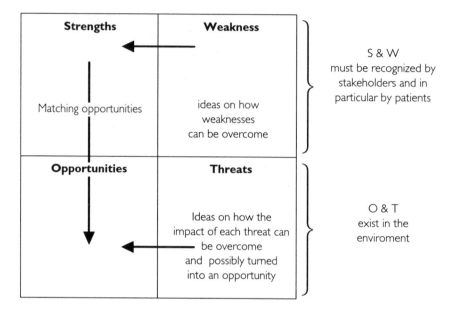

Figure 7.2:   The patient oriented SWOT

DEVELOPING A VISION AND A MISSION FOR THE PRACTICE

A considerable amount of recent management research has highlighted the importance of vision and mission statements and their role in providing staff with a sense of direction and purpose. In general practice, the overall statement of vision would be concerned with an expression of the sort of practice that the partners are trying to create in the medium to long term. An obvious example of this would be that of a practice which has the strongest reputation locally for the quality of patient care and up-to-date facilities (the position of the vision within the planning hierarchy is illustrated in Figure 7.3). You might therefore ask yourself the following question: To what extent is there currently a *shared* and *explicit* vision amongst the partners of the sort of practice that we are trying to develop?

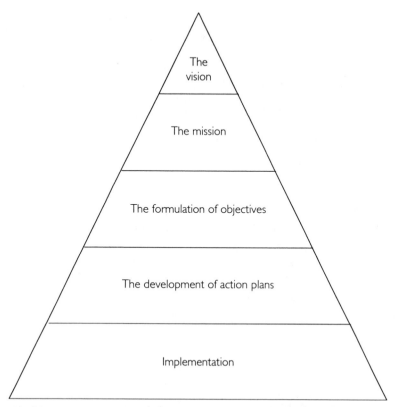

The vision

The mission

The formulation of objectives

The development of action plans

Implementation

Figure 7.3:   The planning hierarchy

In the majority of practices that we have come across, there appears to have been relatively little detailed thought or discussion amongst the partners of this sort of issue, with the partners having concentrated instead upon a whole series of shorter-term issues within the practice. It is, however a fundamental part of the planning process, since it represents a collective statement of what in the long-term you are really trying to achieve.

The significance of a shared vision needs to be seen therefore in terms of the broad framework that it is capable of providing and the influence that this should then have both upon the subsequent mission statement and the sorts of objectives that are set.

Recognizing this, reflect again on the question above and consider raising it at the next partners' meeting with a view to getting an explicit statement of the sort of practice that you are collectively trying to create. To help with this, you might usefully debate the three questions below:

1. What do we want the practice to be like and known for in, say, five years time? (In answering this, take into account not just medical issues and the reputation, but also the size of the practice and its location)

2. How realistic is this vision?

3. What do we need to do if we are to translate this vision into reality?

Having established the vision, you can then move on to the development of the mission statement. A mission statement represents a statement of core values and again, is part of the framework within which the plans are prepared. It is for this reason that at least one commentator has referred to the mission as 'an invisible hand' which guides staff to work in particular ways. There are numerous examples of good mission statements outside general practice, two of which are illustrated in Box 7.3.

Having looked at many hundreds of mission statements over the past few years – some of which have been good, some bad, and others simply a tribute to the ability of the managers to fantasize – there are several points which are worth keeping in mind when developing a mission statement for your practice. They include:

- make sure that it gives a general direction and encompasses key values, it should not include goals or actions;

- keep it short, otherwise staff will probably never read it, far less remember it or really understand it;

- make sure that it focuses upon fundamental issues and reflects core practice values that will neither need changing nor be changed every six months or so;

- make sure that it is believable and is not made up of a series of unrealistic 'wish' statements;

- make sure that it is exciting and inspirational;

- make sure that it is communicated and explained to staff throughout the practice and that a copy is posted in a prominent position in the waiting room;

- recognize that although a first draft can be prepared by one person, the creation of one that is truly worthwhile can only be done as the result of a detailed discussion of practice values and aspirations.

Box 7.3:   Mission statements

Sainsbury's mission statement:

- To discharge the responsibility as leaders in our trade by acting with complete integrity, by carrying out our work to the highest standards, and by contributing to the public good and to the quality of life in the community.

- To provide unrivalled value to our customers in the quality of the goods we sell, in the competitiveness of our prices and in the choice we offer.

- In our stores, to achieve the highest standards of cleanliness and hygiene, efficiency of operation, convenience and customer service, and thereby create as attractive and friendly a shopping environment as possible.

- To offer our staff outstanding opportunities in terms of personal career development and in remuneration relative to other companies in the same market, practising always a concern for the welfare of every individual.

- To generate sufficient profit to finance continual improvement and growth of the business whilst providing our shareholders with an excellent return on their investment.

Marks and Spencer's mission is broadly similar:

- To offer our customers a selective range of high quality, well designed and attractive merchandise at reasonable prices.

- To encourage our suppliers to use the most modern and efficient techniques of production and quality control dictated by the latest discoveries in science and technology.

- With the co-operation of our suppliers, to ensure the highest standards of quality control.

- To plan the expansion of our stores for the better display of a widening range of goods (and) for the convenience of our customers.

- To simplify operating procedures so that our business is carried on in the most efficient manner.

- To foster good human relations with customers, suppliers and staff.

Putting these guidelines into practice involves focusing upon two interrelated dimensions: the *patient related issues* (ie what patients' needs do we intend meeting and where?) and the *key values* (ie what core values, such as quality and levels of patient service, will it encompass and which we are simply not prepared to compromise on?), both of which are encompassed in a mission statement that we came across recently:

> 'As a practice, our mission is to provide our patients with the highest levels of health care at all times by understanding, anticipating and responding to their full range of medical needs, providing a highly accessible service that is of the highest quality, and contributing wherever possible to the improvement of the social fabric of the community by means of a programme of health education and the influence of opinion leaders.'

This statement, which was developed by the partners and staff of a practice in the East Midlands, incorporates a number of the guidelines that we highlighted earlier. Whilst scope exists for some improvement, it has so far proved to be of enormous value within the practice in that it has underlined the sorts of values that are seen to be at the heart of the practice.

With this discussion in mind, consider the following questions:

- Does your practice have a mission statement already? If so, does it reflect the sorts of guidelines that we referred to earlier and incorporate the values that are at the heart of the practice, or is it simply empty rhetoric?

- If the practice does not yet have a mission statement, what value do you think might be gained from developing one?

STEP TWO

Where do we want to go?

How to set worthwhile objectives
To be effective, a planning system must be goal driven. The setting of clear and meaningful objectives is therefore a key step in the marketing planning process, since unless it is carried out effectively, everything that follows will lack focus and cohesion. The purpose of setting objectives is therefore to provide the practice with a sense of direction. In addition, however, they can be used as a basis for motivation as well as a benchmark against which performance and effectiveness can subsequently be measured.

The ten guidelines for setting worthwhile and meaningful objectives are straightforward and are listed in Box 7.4.

Against the background of these guidelines, consider the following questions:

- What are the practice's short-term and long-term objectives currently?

- To what extent do the practice's objectives conform to the ten guidelines in Box 7.4?

- How often are the objectives reviewed in detail?

Box 7.4:   The ten guidelines for worthwhile objectives

Objectives need to be:

1. Hierarchical, from the most important to the least important;

2. Quantifiable, allowing performance against target to be measured at a later stage;

3. Limited in number and concentrated on the most important areas (If you set a large number of objectives, it is likely that not only will you lose sight of at least some of them, but that you will make the process of developing a strategy capable of achieving all of them unnecessarily difficult);

4. Realistic and a true reflection of the practice's strengths, the environmental opportunities, your contractual obligations, and the level of practice capability rather than a series of wishful thoughts;

5. Consistent rather than mutually incompatible;

6. Related to well-defined time periods;

7. Stated explicitly with no scope for ambiguity;

8. Based upon the practice's strengths and designed to help overcome weaknesses;

9. Communicated to staff throughout the practice and the implications for how they operate explained to them;

10. A reflection of the various elements of your mission statement.

- How often and in what detail is performance against objectives measured?

- How much detailed thought is given to the process of developing and implementing the actions needed to achieve these objectives?

IDENTIFYING THE AREAS THAT YOUR OBJECTIVES SHOULD COVER

In setting the objectives for the practice, you need to aim for a balance between several areas such as:

- the partners' expectations;

- FHSA demands;

- the expectations and needs of staff;

- the issues associated with the long term development of the practice, its premises and equipment;

- patients' expectations of the quality of care and levels of service they will receive.

Although this is not an exhaustive list, it provides a useful start to identifying the types of objectives that you might need to consider developing. You should therefore take each of these in turn and list the key points which need to be examined. In the case of patients, for example, you might single out issues such as average waiting times, the length of the consultation, out-of-hours appointments and so on. Under the heading of FHSA demands, you might include the achievement of the upper target for vaccinations and immunizations, whilst staff related issues might include levels of training, and so on. Having identified the key issues under each of these and any other headings that you see to be important, you can then begin the process of refining the list of objectives, making them more specific and attaching timescales so that some will be essentially short term (all reception staff to have reached a pre-determined level of IT capability within twelve months) whilst others, such as the complete refurbishment of the practice's premises, will take longer.

Having done this, you can begin reviewing the objectives with a view to seeing which, if any, are unrealistic either in terms of their magnitude (in other words, they are simply too ambitious) or that are unlikely to be achieved in the short term but can be achieved over a slightly longer period. In doing this, you are trying to ascertain the nature and significance of any shortfalls or gaps that exist between the partners' expectations and the ability of partners and staff throughout the practice to meet these expectations. With this information, you can either modify the objective or increase the degree of attention and the resources paid to its achievement.

As an example of such gap analysis, consider the dual objective of reducing average waiting times while increasing the length of the consultation periods. By giving detailed thought to what is likely to be involved in achieving this, it may become apparent that it can be achieved only partially by increasing appointment hours and that a more radical step is needed if it is to be met completely. This might include either the appointment of a new doctor or each of the current GPs taking an additional surgery each week. Weighing up the alternatives, you may then decide that whilst the objective is laudable, the practice is simply not willing to make the sorts of changes that would be needed for it to be achieved. If this is the case, you need to go back and either modify the objective or cross it out altogether.

STEP THREE

How are we going to get there?

Developing the action plans that will work
Once your short- and long-term objectives are identified, you are then in a position to begin developing action plans. In doing this, you often need to be very specific and to pay ample attention, not just to the question of what needs to be done, but also to who is to be responsible for each element and what intermediate measures on checks on performance are needed; a framework for this appears in Box 7.5.

Implementation is often the most difficult part of the planning process, since it is all too easy to be side-tracked by the sheer pressure of day-to-day activities. In the light of this, you need to give thought to three questions:

1. Who within the practice is to be responsible for driving the plan?

2. How often do you intend holding review meeting to check on the progress being made and whether any corrective action is needed?

3. What sort of feedback are you going to give the staff on how well or badly the plan's implementation is proving to be?

Box 7.5:   The action planning framework

Objectives	Actions needed to achieve these objectives	Allocation of responsibilities	Intermediate performance measures
Short term • • • • Long term • • • •			

The question of who is to drive the plan is important, since whoever takes on the responsibility for this has to recognize from the outset that much of the plan's subsequent success will depend upon how well the job is done. It is therefore essential that in deciding who is to do this, that:

- they are fully committed to the plan and understand each of its elements in detail;

- they have the authority and enthusiasm to make sure that no one loses sight of what the plan involves and what their contribution to its implementation involves.

HOW LONG SHOULD THE PLAN BE?

Perhaps the most frequently asked question in discussing marketing plans with GPs concerns the plan's length. Our advice is always the same: keep the plan as short, straightforward and simple as possible and, above all, make sure that it is capable of being used as a *working document*. Secondly, having written it, do not make the mistake of filing it or assuming that its implementation will take place as if by magic. To say whether it should be ten pages or 20 is impossible. Instead, we would remind you again of the benefits of the planning process (assuming, of course, that it has been done properly) in that it forces you to look not just at the detail of the practice's strengths and weaknesses, but also at the environment and the objectives that you intend pursuing. We would also point out the way in which planning can clarify a considerable number of issues by bringing them into sharper focus and again, assuming that it has been done properly, lead to better patterns of communication, understanding and commitment throughout the practice. Having said all of this, the answer to the question of length has to be that it is not particularly important, but that the two overriding characteristics of worthwhile plans are, first, that they are used as working documents and reflect a planning culture in which full recognition is given to the benefits of the various stages of the analysis and so on, and second, that it helps you to achieve objectives that are seen within the practice to be worthwhile.

THE NINE PLANNING PITFALLS TO AVOID

In working with a variety of practices and helping the partners to develop marketing plans, we have encountered a number of common planning difficulties which, once you are aware of them, are relatively easy to overcome. They are:

1. A tendency to assume that budgeting and planning are one and the same thing; they are not.

2. The development of too many and unrealistically ambitious objectives.

3. An unclear vision of the sort of practice that the partners are trying to develop.

4. An emphasis upon analysis rather than decisions and implementation.

5. Poor internal communications with the result that levels of staff understanding and commitment to the plan are less than they should be.

6. Seeing planning as a ritual rather than an activity which is capable of making a real contribution to the development of the practice.

7. Inadequate resourcing and poor implementation procedures.

8. Failing to allocate responsibilities sufficiently clearly.

9. Poor monitoring, feedback and control.

To sum up, it should be apparent that there is a set of simple guidelines for effective planning. These include the need to:

- treat the plan as a working document (do not file it);

- make it realistic and based on the practice's real strengths and weaknesses;

- keep it simple and user friendly;

- make sure that it reflects opportunities and comes to terms with any threats that exist or seem likely to emerge;

- ensure that it reflects a long-term vision of the sort of practice you are trying to create;

- make sure that it improves teamworking and commitment;

- see it as an opportunity to question the conventional wisdom;

- allocate responsibilities clearly;

- make sure the timescales are realistic;

- monitor performance and do not be afraid to take corrective action where it is needed;

- emphasize communication by getting others involved from the outset – osmosis is only rarely a useful or adequate method of communication;

- make sure that the plan can be and is implemented.

SUMMARY

Within this chapter, we have focused upon the three principal steps of the planning process. Insofar as it is possible to pick out the elements that characterize effective planning, there would have to be the involvement and commitment of staff at all levels of the practice, both to the development and to the implementation of the plan. Without this, any attempt at planning is likely to prove to be of little real value. Recognizing this, there are three final guidelines which you need to bear in mind:

1. Avoid the ivory tower syndrome in which the senior partner develops the plan in isolation, presents it to the partners and staff, and then expects a full-blooded commitment to its implementation.

2. Make sure that staff throughout the practice are involved in the process from as early a stage as possible and are then made fully aware of the contribution that is expected of them in its implementation.

3. Always provide feedback on how well or how badly the practice is performing, highlighting what the next stage of development will be.

8

Using the marketing audit to assess the true level of practice capability: revisiting your strengths and weaknesses

Having read this chapter, you should:

- understand the nature and role of the marketing audit;
- be aware of the audit's components;
- understand how to conduct a marketing audit.

One of the biggest and most common problems faced by organizations, regardless of their type and size, is that plans all too often fail to come to fruition. There are several explanations for this, the most widespread of which are that the objectives set are too ambitious, too little thought is given to the activities needed to achieve the plan, and, faced with day-to-day pressures, staff lose sight of what they are trying to achieve. Because of this, and as we pointed out in Chapters six and seven, effective marketing planning must be based upon a clear statement of *realistic* objectives and a detailed understanding of what the practice is really *capable* of achieving. Although there are several ways in which the practice's capability can be measured, one of the most useful and straightforward tools for this is the *marketing audit* which requires you to focus upon a series of dimensions, such as the practice strategy, its systems and the levels of productivity, with a view to revealing in detail the practice's strength and weakness.

Although the idea of looking at the practice's strengths, weaknesses, opportunities and threats was discussed in Chapter seven, our experience has shown that GPs often produce better and more tightly focused SWOT analyses if they are faced with a framework of questions rather than having to generate them themselves. It is this which, therefore, represents the real rationale for this chapter.

THE COMPONENTS OF THE AUDIT

The marketing audit involves looking in detail at six areas:

1. *The environment:* how are environmental forces developing currently and how are they likely to change in the short-term and the long-term?

2. *The practice strategy:* how well formulated are the objectives and the strategy and how well suited are they to the current and future environments?

3. *The organization:* how capable is the practice of implementing any action plans that are developed?

4. *The systems:* how appropriate and effective are the practice's systems for planning and control?

5. *Productivity:* how cost-effective are the different areas of the practice?

6. *Facilities and resources:* how well suited are the practice's facilities to what you are trying to achieve?

Quite deliberately, the audit that we discuss here is not all embracing, but is instead designed to encourage you to think about specific aspects of the practice. Supplementary questions can therefore be added to make it more directly relevant to an individual practice. In working your way through the six sections above, you should therefore continually pose two fundamental questions:

1. What are the implications of my answer for the practice?

2. What are we/am I going to do about these implications?

For the results of the audit to be worthwhile, a few simple rules need to be kept in mind, including:

1. The process must be comprehensive and cover all parts of the practice rather than just a few known trouble spots;

2. It must be systematic and follow an orderly sequence of steps;

3 It must be independent and not influenced by personal feelings, relationships or preconceived notions.

WHO SHOULD CONDUCT THE AUDIT?

Of the several options open to you, the first, which is also the cheapest and often the fastest, involves the practice manager taking on the responsibility for conducting the audit. There are, however, potential disadvantages in this in that, with the best will in the world, the practice manager may not necessarily be totally objective. Because of this, within a number of the practices that we have dealt with, we have established a small audit task force consisting of the practice manager, one of the partners, and one or two other staff. By doing this, awkward questions are more likely to be addressed and a generally broader perspective brought to the exercise.

As you complete each section of the audit, you need to assess the implications of your answers and identify the sorts of actions and responses that they demand of the practice; the framework for this is drawn up in Box 8.1, which appears at the end of the chapter. As an example, if the strategy audit suggests that the practice's objectives are either not clearly stated or sufficiently well communicated to the staff throughout the practice, the steps to correct this need to be spelled out, responsibilities allocated, acted upon and a reporting back date agreed. Equally, if the productivity audit suggests that certain areas have cost levels that are too high, again an action plan to deal with this needs to be developed.

Having completed all six sections, the findings can then be pulled together in the form of the sort of SWOT (Strengths, Weaknesses, Opportunities and Threats) framework that we discussed in Chapter seven, with extensive thought being given to the actions needed to exploit strengths, convert any weaknesses to strengths, and threats to possible opportunities.

The environmental audit

- What effect will forecasted trends in the size, age distribution and regional distribution of the population have on the practice?

- What changes in attitude are taking place amongst the public towards medical practices?

- What changes are taking place in consumers' lifestyles and values that will have a bearing on our patient groups?

- How do our current patients perceive and rate the practice?

- In what ways are our patients' expectations changing?

- What new clinics are likely to be required over the next few years?

- To what extent are our patients' current expectations being met?

- How might patients best be categorized (eg young/old, regular/occasional visitors to the surgery)? What are the expected rates of growth of each of these categories?

- How are other practices nearby perceived?

- How do other practices operate and what might we learn from them?

- How do different groups of patients appear to make their choice of doctor and practice?

- How are the expectations of external bodies (eg FHSA) likely to change over the next few years?

The strategy audit

- Are the practice's short-term and long-term objectives sufficiently clearly stated?

- Are they understood by everyone in the practice?

- Is there general agreement on their validity?

- Do the objectives provide sufficient guidance for planning and control purposes?

- Are the objectives appropriate given the demands of patients and the external environment?

- Is there a well-formulated practice strategy?

- If so, are staff aware of the strategy and the nature of the contribution that they are expected to make to it?

- Have sufficient resources been optimally allocated across the various patient groups?

- Are there any new services or clinics that we might offer?

- Are there any services or clinics that might benefit from minor or major changes being made to them?

- Are there any services or clinics that we offer currently which should be dropped?

- What are the practice's promotional objectives?

- Is there a well-conceived publicity programme?

The organizational audit

- Is there someone who has direct responsibility for planning and monitoring performance? If so, does this person have adequate authority?

- Are responsibilities within the practice clearly spelled out and understood?

- Are the lines of communication and working relations between staff operating as effectively as they might?

- Are lines of authority within the practice clearly spelled out?

- Are there any individuals within the practice who need more training, motivation, supervision or evaluation?

- Do staff evaluations take place regularly?

- Is there sufficient teamworking?

- What conflicts exist within the practice?

- Do you hold regular brainstorming sessions in order to identify how levels of patient service might be improved?

- Is the task of motivation taken sufficiently seriously or is it assumed that all staff will always be well motivated?

- Are briefing and feedback sessions held on a regular basis?

- Is an open managerial style in operation?

The systems audit

- Is the system for identifying what is happening outside the practice and which is of potential significance working effectively?

- Is the planning system well conceived and effective?

- Are realistic targets set for staff?

- Is there an adequate monitoring system in place so that performance is measured objectively?

- Are the control procedures (monthly and quarterly) to ensure that the annual plan objectives are met operating effectively?

- Is sufficient provision made to monitor, analyse and evaluate the costs of various services?

- Is the practice organized to ensure that new ideas are generated and evaluated?

- What mechanisms exist to ensure that levels of patient satisfaction are being monitored?

- Are the computer systems working effectively and are they adequate for the ways in which the practice will probably develop?

The productivity audit

- What formal mechanisms exist to ensure that all cost areas are reviewed on a regular basis?

- Do any activities appear to have excessive costs?

- What steps are being taken to:
  (i) control costs
  (ii) reduce costs?

- Are brainstorming sessions held on a regular basis in order to identify how levels of productivity might possibly be improved?

- Do there appear to be any unnecessary procedures or processes within the practice?

- Are there any procedures or processes that might usefully be modified?

The facilities and resources audit

- How do patients view our physical premises?

- What changes do we need to make to improve them?

- Is the practice adequately resourced to achieve the objectives that have been set?

Box 8.1:   The findings and implications of the marketing audit

Findings	The implications	Actions required
The environmental audit • • • •		
The strategy audit • • • •		
The organizational audit • • • •		
The systems audit • • • •		
The productivity audit • • • •		
The facilities and resources audit • • • •		

- In which areas is further investment needed?

- What obstacles do patients experience in visiting the surgery?

SUMMARY

Having conducted the audit, there are several questions which need to be considered.

- What picture of the practice emerges?

- What areas within the practice do we need to pay attention to in the short-term and in the long-term?

- What courses of action do we need to take?

- Who is to be given the responsibility for each of these?

- What are the resource implications of any changes that are needed?

One further question that needs to be raised concerns the issue of cause and effect. Where something has gone wrong or levels of performance are not as high as they might or should be, you need to spend time identifying why this has happened and who is primarily responsible. In doing this, the purpose is not to point the finger of blame but instead is designed to highlight the nature of any training that might be needed to overcome a skills problem and/or whether a change in the allocation of responsibilities might be appropriate.

9

Developing the practice's marketing mix

Having read this chapter, you should:

- understand the various elements that make up the marketing mix;
- have an appreciation of the nature and significance of the role played by the mix within the marketing process and of the ways in which managing the mix is capable of affecting the demand of the practice's services.

We first made reference to the marketing mix in Chapter two, suggesting that it consists of seven dimensions – the product/service, promotion, place, price, people, process management and physical elements. Together, these elements, which are sometimes referred to as the 7Ps, make up the marketing tool kit that is used to shape the profile of the practice that is presented to the world.

Here we focus upon each of the seven elements in turn and then discuss how they can be brought together in the form of a coherent marketing programme and action plan.

THE PRODUCT/SERVICE

Almost invariably, the starting point for any discussion of the marketing mix has to be the product or service offered, since it is this which provides the basis for virtually all other marketing decisions. In the case of general practice, the 'product' that patients receive is made up of three distinct dimensions: the product's attributes, its benefits, and the nature of the support services; these are illustrated in Figure 9.1.

- *Product attributes* are associated with the core product and are made up of the clinical and medical procedures.

- *Product benefits* are the various elements that patients perceive as meeting their needs – this is sometimes referred to as the 'bundle of satisfaction'; included within this is the perceived and actual effectiveness of the treatment and the reassurance that the patient is given.

- *The support services* consist of all the elements that the practice provides in addition to the core product. These would typically include the appoint-

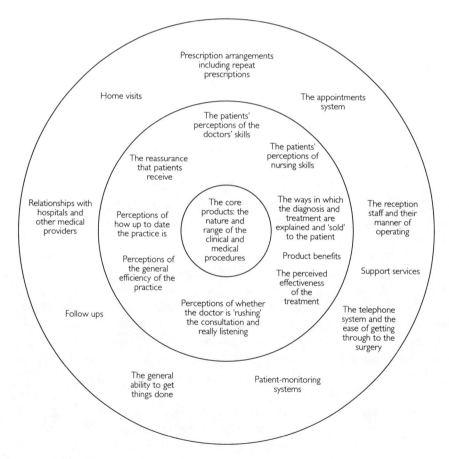

Figure 9.1:   The three levels of the product

ments system, the reception staff and their manner, follow ups, home visits and the relationships that exist between the practice, the hospital and other medical providers.

In looking at Figure 9.1, there are several issues that emerge which are of potentially considerable significance. The first of these is the extent to which the support services are capable of setting the tone for any visit. Following on from this, is the way in which product benefits are influenced not so much by reality, but by patients' perceptions (it might be useful at this stage to refer briefly to our discussion in Chapter three of what patients really want from their doctors see pages 28–30). The third factor is that against this background, medical competence, clinical excellence, levels of expertize and issues of quality are often taken for granted, and in a patient-centred practice in particular are the areas which are least likely to be questioned by patients.

Given the nature of these comments, you might usefully reflect on the points listed in Box 9.1.

In answering the final question posed in Box 9.1, there are two models, the product life cycle and the Ansoff matrix, which are commonly used in marketing and which might be of help in structuring your thinking; these are illustrated in Figures 9.2 and 9.3.

The product life cycle is, in many ways, one of the best known and straightforward of marketing models, and based on the idea that any product or service has a finite life and that during this life there is a need to manage it in particular ways, depending upon the position it has reached.

The majority of the services offered by general practice are, by their very nature, likely to be in the mature phase. However, if the practice is to develop over the next few years and exploit the opportunities now or in the future, you need to consider what additional services might be introduced or, in the case of some of the services offered currently, might be encouraged to grow.

To use the life cycle as a planning tool, you need therefore to begin by positioning each of your products/services on the curve. Having done this, take each of the services in turn and ask whether scope exists for its expansion and growth. If so, think about the sorts of actions that would be needed to do this and what degree of growth might be possible. In the case of minor surgery, for example, considerable opportunities undoubtedly exist in many practices, although in order to realise this potential, a series of possibly significant investment steps and an advancement of skills would be needed. By contrast, many practices could expand the range of health promotion programmes relatively quickly and at a low cost simply by publicizing their existence far more aggressively.

Box 9.1: Checking out your product and support services

The support services

- Is the practice's phone system capable of handling the volume of calls you receive or do patients often find themselves getting an engaged tone?

- Are all the reception staff sufficiently approachable, courteous, helpful and knowledgeable?

- Has the appointments system been designed for the convenience of patients or staff?

- Are the patient-monitoring systems as good as they might be?

- Is there a general culture within the practice of getting things right first time and done on time?

- Are the practice's relationships with hospitals and other medical providers as satisfactory and well-developed as they might be?

- What sorts of problems have been encountered in the system of:
    - (i) follow-ups;
    - (ii) home visits;
    - (iii) repeat prescriptions?

- What scope exists for changes and improvements *for the patient* in each of these areas?

Product benefits: the bundle of satisfactions

- Do you have a detailed understanding of how patients perceive each of the doctors within the practice?

- How do patients appear to perceive the practice in each of the following areas:
    - (i) the nursing skills;
    - (ii) the accuracy of diagnosis;
    - (iii) the explanation and 'selling' of treatments;
    - (iv) the effectiveness of treatments;
    - (v) the general efficiency of the practice;
    - (vi) how up-to-date the practice is;
    - (vii) levels of reassurance?

continued over

Box 9.1:   *continued*

• In what areas does there appear to be scope for improvements? What would be involved in making these improvements and what obstacles would be encountered?

The core product

• What range of clinical and medical services do you offer currently?

• What scope exists for developing each of these services?

• What scope exists for extending these services?

• Are there any services which are offered currently which, for one reason or another, you should consider dropping?

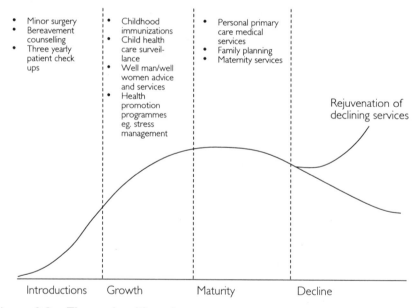

Figure 9.2:   The product life cycle

Where the demand for services appears to have stopped growing and has reached maturity several possibilities exist. The first involves managing the service in such a way that it stays in profitable maturity almost indefinitely by ensuring, for example, that the size of the list remains at least the same and that

Product/services

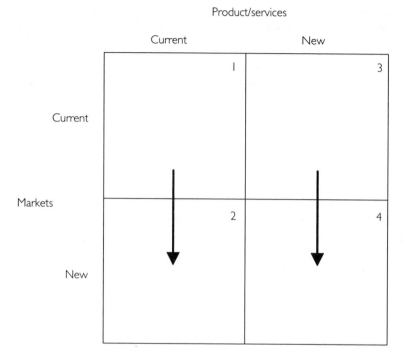

Figure 9.3:   The Ansoff matrix

the amount of primary medical care remains constant. An alternative approach would involve the decision to expand the practice by recruiting a new partner, opening a satellite surgery, or merging with another practice. Above all, of course, you need to guard against the gradual decline of the practice as the result of a series of external changes, such as an increasingly elderly patient profile or a housing redevelopment which leads to people moving away.

Having used the product life cycle as the first step, you need then to think about how the Ansoff matrix can contribute to planning. The matrix, which is illustrated in Figure 9.3, involves looking initially at your existing products/services and markets with a view to identifying the scope that exists for:

1. Extending existing products/services into new or untapped market sectors (eg promoting existing well man and well woman programmes to those patients who you rarely, if ever, see);

2. Developing new products/services for existing markets (eg introducing stress management or bereavement counselling sessions and promoting them to your existing patients);

3. Developing new products/services for new or untapped markets (eg the development of a specialism such as industrial medicine and the pursuit of a contract with local firms as their medical officer).

To use the Ansoff matrix, begin by listing your existing products or services in the top left hand cell of the matrix. Having done this, use brainstorming to generate as many ideas as possible on how all or some of these might be moved into cell three. Try then to name a range of new services that might be set up and offered to your existing markets (cell two) and, in turn, how these might be extended into cell four.

The next stage involves assessing the viability of your ideas by giving detailed thought to what would be involved in developing each product/service and market, whether this would prove to be cost-effective, and indeed whether this would be a development that, individually, the partners would welcome. In doing this, there is a further framework that can be of help; this is illustrated in Figure 9.4 and Box 9.2.

The practice's ability/
willingness to service areas of
specific need effectively

	High	Low
High	Money makers	Political hot potatoes
Patients' needs and their match with levels and availability of funding support	Wasted efforts	Back drawer items
Low		

Figure 9.4: The practice's ability/willingness to service areas of specific need effectively

Box 9.2: Patient need and funding support

Areas of patient need	The match between areas of patient need and the levels and availability of funding support	Willingness/ability of the practice to service each area of patient need
•	High/Low*	High/Low*
•	High/Low*	High/Low*
•	High/Low*	High/Low*
•	High/Low*	High/Low*
•	High/Low*	High/Low*
•	High/Low*	High/Low*
•	High/Low*	High/Low*
•	High/Low*	High/Low*

*delete as applicable

To use the matrix in Figure 9.4, you need to begin by using the first column of the table in Box 9.2 to list as many areas of patient need as possible. Having done this, complete the second column which is concerned with the levels and availability of funding support, then complete the third column which deals with the practice's ability/willingness to service effectively each of these areas of patient need.

Finally, enter each of the areas in the appropriate cells of the matrix in Figure 9.4. From the picture that emerges, you should then be in a position to identify those areas in which you might usefully concentrate some of the practice's future energies and those from which you might possibly either withdraw or at least reduce your focus. In the case of the money makers, for example, there is an obvious incentive to increase practice effort. For the political hot potatoes, detailed thought needs to be given to the various ways in which practice efforts might possibly be channelled in these directions; the obvious area, of course, from which at least some of this resource might come, is the wasted effort cell.

Equally, serious thought needs to be given to the future of those activities which appear in the back drawer cell.

PROMOTION

Although doctors are not allowed to advertize, there are several ways in which the practice can be promoted. However, before discussing some of the ways in which this might be done, you need to give thought to the sort of image that you would like to create for the practice.

Is it, for example, that of a highly innovative, thrusting, dynamic and high-tech partnership or one that is wedded to traditional values? The answer to this will depend in part upon the types of partners you have, but also upon the types of patients on your list. In some instances, of course, patients might well be disconcerted by what they see to be an overly modern and aggressive approach to health care.

In debating how you will manage this part of the marketing mix, you should begin by considering four questions:

1. What sort of image does the practice have currently?

2. What sort of image do you, as doctors, want to create?

3. What sort of image do your patients want and what will they feel most comfortable with?

4. What sorts of images do other practices locally have?

Patients build up an image of a practice in a wide variety of ways. Typically this includes the age and manner of the doctors, the type and location of the premises, the ways in which the telephone is answered, the reception staff, the waiting area, the consulting room, the look of the equipment, letters and letter headings, word of mouth, the doctors' cars, and so on. Recognition of this should give you a better understanding of the number of areas to which you will have to pay attention if you decide to make any real change to the image that exists currently. In some cases, of course, some of the areas that we have identified can be changed at relatively low cost; the practice leaflets and the letter headings are obvious examples. In other cases, however, changes will either be far more difficult, time-consuming and expensive, or simply not open to modification; the age and manner of doctors tend to spring to mind as the most obvious examples of the sorts of constraints which you would have to work around.

It should be apparent from this discussion that there is probably very little that can be gained from playing around with just one or two promotional elements, and that a far more focused effort is likely to be needed. Box 9.3 should help in achieving this.

Box 9.3:   The promotion check-up checklist

- What overall image does the practice have currently?
- What image do you want to create?
- How big a shift is going to be required in order to achieve this?
- In what ways might each of the promotional elements contribute to this new image?
- How big is the promotional budget for the next 12 months?
- Who will have the responsibility for developing and implementing the new image?
- What design skills do you have within the practice? (Never forget that highly developed design skills are relatively rare and that you will probably save a lot of time and effort by going to a design shop at the outset rather than trying to do it yourself or letting one of the reception staff do it 'because she's creative').

It is worthwhile at this point to spend some time thinking about the complete spectrum of factors that contribute to the practice's image; in addition to those that we identified at an earlier stage in this section, there is of course:

* the annual report;

* the practice leaflets;

* practice newsletters;

* the entry in the Yellow Pages;

* letters to patients (not just the letter heads and style of the letter, but also the type of paper and envelopes).

In each case, try to be objective by standing to one side and asking yourself what you would think of each of these if you were looking at them for the first time. Having done this, consider how each one might be improved (never be afraid to look at what other GPs and other professionals such as solicitors, accountants, vets and so on are doing). Try also a brainstorming session where you could raise, for example, the question of the scope that exists for using the records system to target certain groups of patients with a personal letter to tell them about a particularly relevant service, or sending cards to newly born babies.

   When concentrating upon developing the action plan that will help achieve and reinforce the image that you are trying to create never lose sight of three golden rules:

1. Have a clear 'house style' which is used on all forms of promotion;

2. Keep messages simple;

3. Always emphasize the benefits that patients will receive.

With these in mind, you can start to prepare the sort of action plan that appears in Box 9.4.

Box 9.4:   The promotion action plan

The image that we want to create is that of a practice which is . . . .

The ways in which we will do this include:

	Key messages	Timing	Responsibility
• Practice leaflets			
• The Yellow Pages			
• The annual report			
• Letters to the patients			
• Notices in the waiting room			
• The practice newsletter			
• What staff tell patients			
• The layout and decor of the waiting room			
•			
•			

PLACE AND THE PHYSICAL ELEMENTS

For these purposes, the place and physical elements of the practice's marketing mix can be discussed in tandem, since they are concerned with three interrelated factors: the location of the practice; its accessibility and its general ambience and the sorts of messages that patients receive from it both internally and externally.

In evaluating this part of the mix, you should therefore give consideration to several questions, including:

1. How conveniently is the surgery located? (Although in the short-term you might not be able to change the location, this is almost certain to be a possibility in the longer term.)

2. Is there a need for a small, satellite surgery on two or three occasions each week?

3. How accessible does the appointments system make the practice?

4. How often do appointments run late (and how many patients are affected)?

5. What does the design, layout, cleanliness and warmth of the waiting room say about the practice?

6. Are there sufficient distractions for patients while they are waiting? Eg toys for children, music, and health promotion videos.

7. How does it compare with the waiting room of other surgeries, and indeed of the waiting areas in solicitors' and accountants' offices?

8. Would you feel comfortable sitting in the waiting room as it is laid out currently?

PRICE

In any discussion of the practice marketing mix, price often proves to be the most difficult to come to terms with. There are several reasons for this, although the most obvious stems from the way in which patients do not pay for their treatment at the time or point of delivery, but instead via the tax mechanism. Because of this, doctors are faced with having to satisfy two groups: the patients who represents the health care consumer, and the FHSA which represents the health care customer.

The result of this and of the ways in which the health service has developed, is that patients' expectations often bear little real relation to the cost of the treatment with the consequent danger of the system either being under-valued or misused. From the viewpoint of the FHSA (that is, the customer rather than the consumer), the issue of value for money takes on an infinitely greater importance. Because of this, the FHSA has a degree of flexibility and discretion in how it responds to particular initiatives, something which is most obviously seen in their decision on whether to fund particular health promotion programmes. In looking at the price element of the mix, it is perhaps easier therefore to focus upon issues of cost and in particular just how cost-effective each element of the practice is. Given this, how would you answer the following?

•   How detailed is our understanding of the costs of each major dimension of the practice?

- Are there any areas in which costs are unnecessarily high?

- In what ways and in what areas might we be more cost effective?

PEOPLE

In our earlier discussion of the product/service component of the mix, we highlighted the significance of patient perception and how this is influenced by the manner, behaviour and responses not just of the doctor, but also of the nursing and reception staff. Because of this, the effective management of the people element has to be seen as a crucial part of the practice's marketing effort, since it is capable of making or breaking the programme. Consider therefore, the following questions:

Non-medical staff

- How rigorous is your selection procedure for non-medical staff?

- What initial and subsequent training do they receive?

- Are the staff encouraged to work in teams and do these teams work effectively?

- Do you encourage or demand a certain standard of dress? Do you have a uniform that non-medical staff are required to wear?

- What effort has gone into customer care training?

- What problems do you appear to have amongst your non-medical staff?

- What are working relationships like?

- Are there sufficient non-medical staff of the right sort and with the right skills to enable you to achieve the practice objectives?

Medical staff

- Are the medical staff fully up-to-date with medical and administrative procedures?

- Have they been properly trained in how to handle patients effectively or do they just rely upon common sense? (Never forget that common sense is an all too rare commodity.)

- What additional medical and non-medical training will they require over the next few years?

- Are working relationships between the medical staff satisfactory?

- Are the working relationships between the medical and the non-medical staff as effective as they might be?

Looking at the practice overall:

- Do you have the right blend of skills and experience for what is being demanded of general practice in the 1990s?

- What are the levels of motivation and morale like?

In the light of your answers to these questions, you should be in a better position to begin the process of identifying in greater detail the sorts of skills and knowledge gaps that exist and which are likely to affect the patient experience and hence their perceptions of the practice.

PROCESS MANAGEMENT

The final part of the mix is concerned with the ways in which patients and information are handled. Although we have already made a number of references to issues such as how patients are dealt with, both by the reception and the medical staff, it is worth posing just a few more questions. How, for example, are patients addressed? Is it in a relatively formal way or, as we came across in one practice, as 'Luv' or 'Duck' and on one memorable occasion as 'Mate'? How are patients summoned by the doctor? Is it with a buzzer, is it by the doctor shouting down the corridor 'Next!', or is it by a member of the reception staff? Whichever approach is used, think clearly about how you would feel if you were the patient in these circumstances.

The second dimension of process management is concerned with the ways in which the various systems within the practice operate including the patients' record systems, recall procedures, and the accuracy of the consultation recording process. The questions that you should therefore consider under this heading include:

- Are we making as much use of information technology as we might or should?

- How might the various systems be developed?

- What information do we need to make the practice work more effectively and deliver a higher level of patient service?

- Do we have a clear idea of how we might do this?

DEVELOPING THE ACTION PLAN

Against the background of your answers to the questions posed so far, you should now be in a position to begin the process of pulling together the individual elements of the marketing mix in the form of an action plan; a framework to help with this appears in Box 9.5. To complete the framework, start by identifying your objectives under each of the headings of the marketing mix. Then move on to list, in as much detail as possible, the action steps that will need to be taken in order to achieve the objectives. However, recognizing that not every objective or action is of equal importance or equally pressing, try to assess the degree of priority and the timescales over which the various courses of action should take place. From here, move on to quantify the broad levels of costs that will be incurred and then, finally, begin the process of allocating responsibilities.

FOCUSING THE MARKETING EFFORT

As in life generally, so it is that in marketing it is only rarely possible to be all things to all people. Because of this, any marketing programme for the practice needs to reflect the different types of patient on your list by being tailored to a variety of patient needs and expectations. There are various ways in which this can be done including categorizing (segmenting) patients on the basis of factors such as:

- age

- sex

Box 9.5:   The marketing mix action planning framework

	Objectives	Summary of actions needed to achieve the objectives	Degree of priority	Time scales	Costs	Responsibilities
Product/ service						
Promotion						
Place/physical elements						
Price						
People						
Process management						

- family size
- family type (eg single parent, sole survivor, married with two young children and so on)
- social class, lifestyle and culture
- general patterns of health and usage levels of the practice
- benefits required (eg counselling, treatment for a specific illness, long term care, and so on)
- urban/rural dwellers
- ethnic origin and/or religion
- attitudes to medical treatment (eg high dependency, sceptical, a necessity, etc.)

- smokers and non smokers

- types of illness and treatment needed

- expectations of the practice.

Although we are not arguing that all of these approaches to segmenting the patient list should be used, you need to go through each of them and decide which are the most relevant for your practice. Having done this, you can then begin thinking about how the marketing effort might be tailored to each of the principal groups.

In a broader sense, understanding the structure of your patient list and how it is changing can provide general insights into how the practice might best be cultivated and how you should deal with the FHSA.

SUMMARY

In this chapter we have focused upon the nature and importance of the various elements of the marketing mix and highlighted the need to think about ways in which the patient list might be segmented and the marketing effort more readily focused.

Because the mix represents the marketing toolkit used to shape the profile of the practice and determine the face that is presented to the world, the need to ensure that each of the individual elements has been properly developed and pulled together into a coherent whole is paramount. Failure to do this is likely to lead to wasted opportunities and a less than optimal performance. However, the reality in many practices is that varying degrees of attention are paid to the individual elements and rarely is any real attempt made to pull these together in a truly co-ordinated fashion.

Recognizing this, ask yourself the following questions:

- How frequently do we review in detail each of the individual elements of the mix?

- Are the objectives for each element clearly stated?

- Has attention been paid to the development of an explicit marketing mix action plan?

- Is there a clear strategy for pulling together the individual elements in the form of an integrated and fully co-ordinated marketing programme?

- Who has overall responsibility for managing the mix?

- How might the patient list be segmented and the marketing effort more firmly focused? What benefits might this lead to?

10

Setting the standards of customer care: the Blackpool rock phenomenon

Having read this chapter, you should:

* understand what contributes to the total patient experience;

* appreciate the nature of the interaction between medical and non-medical factors;

* be aware of what would be required of your practice if you were to develop an effective customer (patient) care programme.

PATIENTS ARE CUSTOMERS TOO

We commented in Chapter nine that patients generally take their doctor's level of medical competence for granted and that, because of this, the non-medical and support elements of the practice are capable of taking on what some doctors consider to be an unrealistic or unfair degree of importance in determining not just how the practice is perceived generally, but also how good (or bad) the medical dimensions really are. Given this, the argument for focusing upon what we can refer to as the *total patient experience* is inescapable, since it is this which provides the framework for establishing the standards of overall care that the patients – your customers – will perceive that they are getting from the practice.

There are several reasons why the broader aspects of patient/customer care have increased in importance in recent years, although perhaps the most important or most obvious of these are the generally higher expectations of service that now exist and an apparent reduction in the willingness of members of the public to make allowances for what they see to be unreasonable behaviour. Couple this with the public's generally greater willingness to complain and take their custom elsewhere and the arguments for a customer care policy become ever more apparent.

THE BLACKPOOL ROCK PHENOMENON

At the outset, it needs to be emphasized that customer care has moved on considerably from the 'have a nice day' and indeed the 'come back soon, missing you already' approach that characterized numerous care programmes in the early days. Instead, we are concerned here with establishing the standards that will run right the way through the practice (the Blackpool rock phenomenon), and achieving the degree of professionalism across the entire spectrum of the framework within which every aspect of practice-patient interaction takes place.

Any truly effective customer care programme for the practice straddles both the medical and the non-medical dimensions of the practice and it is because of this that you need to begin by considering three fundamental questions:

1. What sort of total experience do you give patients currently?

2. What sort of total experience would you like to give?

3. What are you really capable of delivering?

This reality–intent–capability framework is illustrated in Figure 10.1 and provides a basis for thinking about the size and significance of the gap that exists between intent and capability. There are, of course, numerous factors that can contribute to this gap and having identified its size, significance and the nature of the contributory factors within the practice, thought needs to be given not just to the ways in which the gap might be filled, but also to whether the practice would be willing to allocate the level of resources that would be needed to do this. In making this comment, we have several thoughts in mind, perhaps the most significant of which is that in vitually every practice we have visited, the partners and staff have talked about excellence and providing the very highest levels of patient care. The reality, of course, is that what we can refer to as the Rolls Royce approach is only rarely feasible (or cost-effective) and you need therefore to temper your ideas with a dose of reality.

To help with this, turn to Figure 10.2 and, being brutally honest with yourself, plot where the practice is currently, *and why*. It might be the case, for example that you are in cell two (high standards of medical delivery, but because of

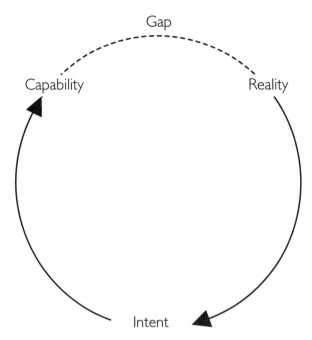

Figure 10.1:   The reality–intent–capability gap

antiquated premises, an archaic telephone system and a dragon of a receptionist, you have relatively poor levels of non-medical support). Having identified the causes in as much detail as possible, you can then begin the detailed analysis of what would be required to move the practice either to another cell (presumably cell one) or to a stronger and more favourable position within the existing cell.

THE LESSONS FROM ELSEWHERE

In our work with a wide variety of different types of organizations, there has proved to be one issue over the past few years that managers have discussed with greater passion than anything else: the standards of customer care and service that their organizations deliver. Almost without exception, every organization we have dealt with, at least in the first instance, has claimed almost unparalleled levels of customer care, something which has led us to conclude that the business world is full of managers with a seemingly infinite capacity for

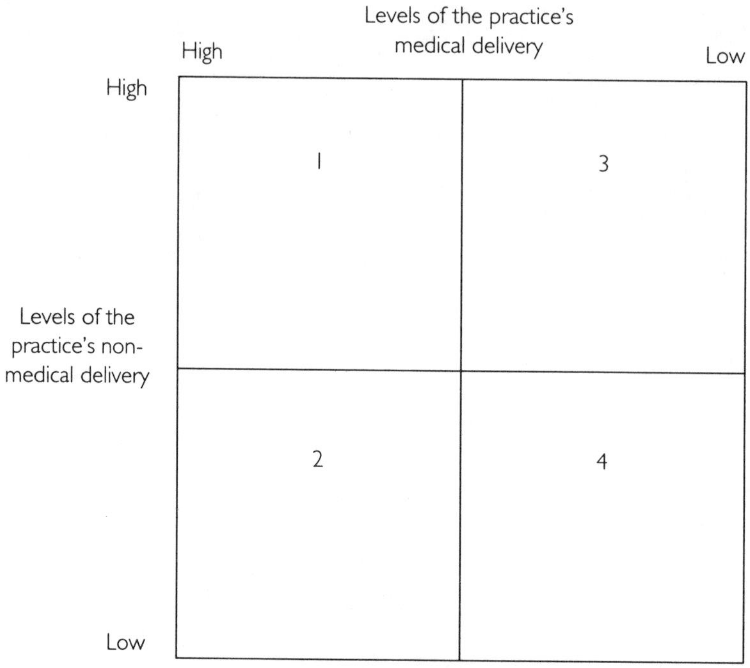

Levels of the practice's
medical delivery

High   Low

Figure 10.2:   The medical/non-medical delivery matrix

self-delusion. There are, of course, exceptions to this and it is to these sorts of organization that we now need to turn with a view to learning what it is that contributes to a truly effective customer care programme. However before doing this, refer to Box 10.1 and recall your experiences in recent weeks as a customer of various types of organization.

Having done this, think about the sort of organizations which consistently achieve high levels of customer care and make a note of what appears to contribute to this. In the case of the high street, for example, organizations such as Marks and Spencer, Sainsbury and McDonald's have been at the forefront in establishing – and maintaining – the levels of service which others simply dream about. In all these cases, the factors which have led to this are straightforward and come down, firstly, to a fundamental belief on the part of senior management in the importance of customer satisfaction, and then, secondly, to the communication of these values to everyone in the organization. High levels of service, and hence satisfaction, therefore becomes the norm in these circumstances rather than the exception.

Box 10.1:   Your experiences of customer care

Think of three organizations that you have dealt with recently.

* What good and bad experiences do you remember?

* Which of these were related to the behaviour of staff and which to the physical aspects of the place such as appearance, cleanliness and atmosphere?

* Did there appear to be any real understanding of 'delight' factors (A 'delight' factor is something that makes you feel especially pleased)?

* When you felt that you were treated either badly or less than very well, what was the effect on you?

* When you have been treated badly or less than perfectly, what efforts have been made to put things right?

* If you have to go back to a place where you have had a poor experience, what attitudes do you take with you?

* Do you think that most people would react to these experiences in much the same way?

By contrast, the major banks seem to operate according to a completely different set of principles altogether. Instead of being open when customers want (9–6 Monday to Saturday and 10–5 on Sundays), opening hours reflect staff demands, banking pressures and historical idiosyncrasies. Equally, at the times of highest demand (12–1.30), staff take lunch breaks and queues form in the branches.

Faced with critical comments such as these, bankers tend to respond by saying, 'But you don't understand our problems'. This sort of response is, however, a nonsense and makes a mockery of any claims of customer service. It is also one of the reasons why the building societies, which do have longer opening hours and manage to present a far friendlier face, consistently score far better than the banks in surveys of customer perceptions of care, approachability and friendliness.

The significance of the role played by senior management in these organizations in establishing the standards of service and customer care should never ever be underestimated, something which has been highlighted by the leading American management guru of the 1980s and early 1990s, Tom Peters. Peters' view is straightforward and unequivocal:

'Claims of quality and customer service mean nothing unless the person at the top of the organization is committed to them 24 hours a day, seven days a week, 52 weeks a year. If you compromise on this even once, you know it, your staff know it and, worst of all, your customers know it.'

The implications of this for general practice and the need for absolute and total commitment on the part of the senior partner to the quality of the total patient experience are (or should be) self-evident.

CUSTOMER CARE IN GENERAL PRACTICE

Relating these points to general practice was first touched upon in Chapter three when we discussed the patient-oriented practice and is not necessarily as difficult to achieve as it might appear at first sight. It does, however, involve running the practice for the convenience of the patients rather than, say, the doctors (this is the equivalent of running the banks for the convenience of the customers rather than the bank staff). In the case of surgery hours, for example, our experiences have shown that in most instances they were established by doctors themselves several years ago and reflect what is convenient for them rather than what is necessarily the most convenient for the patients. In making this comment, we are not arguing for wholesale changes in surgery hours, but rather for an assessment of whether scope exists for small changes that would prove useful from the patients' point of view. Given this, consider the questions in Box 10.2.

In the light of your answers, how do you see the practice and what *overall* level of customer care do you think the practice manages to achieve?

DEVELOPING A PLAN TO IMPROVE CUSTOMER CARE

Once the initial audit is complete, you can turn your attention to the ways in which a programme of customer care can be developed. In doing this, you need to follow a simple four step procedure which is depicted in Figure 10.3.

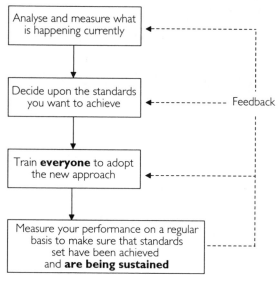

Figure 10.3: Planning customer care

Box 10.2:   The initial customer care audit

- Do those around you always behave professionally towards patients and all other members of staff? If not, what sorts of problems exist, and why?
- What patterns of behaviour in the practice do you consider to be unprofessional?
- What steps have been and are being taken in order to overcome these?
- What do you do in your practice if a patient goes away obviously unhappy because of the ways in which they have been treated?
- What do you know about the reasons why some patients opt to move to another practice?

Do your staff . . .

- always acknowledge patients/visitors as soon as possible and use their name? (In the case of the telephone, you might consider introducing a guideline that the phone will always be answered on or before the third ring between, say 8am and 7pm.)
- welcome the patients and are invariably friendly?
- attempt to reassure them if they are anxious?
- apologize if there is a delay and give an explanation for the delay?
- explain things to them and check that they understand?
- listen to them and check that they understand what you have told them?

Stage 1: The starting point

As a first step, you need to understand in detail how patients (customers) feel about the practice currently, what their expectations are, and the extent to which these expectations are not being met. Although you have already done the initial audit in Box 10.2, and indeed plotted the position of the practice in Figure 10.2, you might find it helpful to run through the following questions:

- In the light of our comments and questions throughout the book, is the practice fundamentally patient or doctor oriented? (In answering this, you might find it useful to refer back to Figure 3.4.)

- Do the partners really accept that the whole image and physical appearance of the practice is important in contributing to customer care?

- Are you clear about what patients really want from the practice?

- What impression do patients get of the practice when they walk through the door?

- Is it likely that they find any aspect of the practice intimidating or off-putting?

- Do you have any formal mechanism currently which allows patients' views to be fed back and influence how the practice operates? (If not, refer back to Chapter four in which we discuss the role of marketing research as a means of measuring levels of patient satisfaction.)

Stage 2: Setting the standards

Appreciating how patients see the practice currently, you need then to address the question of the overall standards of patient care that you want to aim for. In this, we are assuming that the standards of medical care are satisfactory. You should therefore focus upon the range of other factors that influence attitudes and performance such as:

- Is the reception area untidy?

- Are the consulting rooms clean, modern and efficient?

- Is the reception desk a fortress? Does the reception area have distracting or unclear notices?

- Do the reception staff appear welcoming and confident?

- Do the medical staff appear welcoming and confident?

- Do all staff have a good telephone manner and is the phone answered promptly?

- Are appointments easily available and do you have a plan if they are not?

- Do you make sure that all forms of communications with patients are clear and unambiguous?

- How long do patients normally have to wait for an appointment?

- How often do appointments times overrun and by what amount?

- What is the level of availability of vaccines and drugs?

- How accurate is the patients' record system?

- How accessible is the records system?

- How effectively does it work in calling and recalling patients?

- How accessible are doctors both in and out of surgery hours?

In the case of your relationships with external providers, think about the answers to the following questions:

- In general terms, how do your major providers such as hospitals and individual consultants compare with each other in terms of standards, waiting times and access to services?

- Where you have an option, are you encouraging referrals to the best providers?

- How can you bring your needs more fully to the attention of the providers?

- What major strengths and weaknesses does each provider have?

- What are you doing to exploit these strengths?

- Where there are weaknesses, what are you doing to try alternatives?

- Are there opportunities to work more closely with the best providers?

- What are you doing to bring this about?

- What changes do you expect to see amongst providers over the next two years and the next five years? What are the implications of this?

- Who is specifically responsible for assessing your internal data to provide a clear picture of referral patterns?

- What gaps in information do you have?

- What are you doing to set up a system to provide the information?

Stage 3: Planning and implementing the customer care programme

In planning how to implement a new and higher level of customer care, you need to focus upon five areas:

1   Developing a patient-oriented practice mission
Ensure that the practice mission statement includes an explicit expression of the level of patient care you are aiming for. An example of this might be:

> 'As a family practice, our staff are committed to providing the very highest level of medical care for our patients and encouraging the promotion of good health throughout our local community'.

2   Involving the staff at all stages
Having made a statement of the standards you are aiming for, make sure that staff throughout the practice understand this, believe in it and know how it will be achieved. Make sure also that they feel a sense of ownership. In order to achieve this, make sure that as many staff as possible are involved in deciding what should and needs to be done. There are various ways of doing this, eg getting all the staff to complete a questionnaire concerned with what they believe or know of what patients might want from the practice. Other methods for getting ideas involve brainstorming and wide-ranging discussion groups to identify the sorts of changes needed.

3   Defining the requirements of key activities
For certain activities such as answering the telephone, giving instructions, and repeat prescriptions, define *exactly* what is required and develop procedures to ensure that the activity is carried out in a uniform way.

4   Confirm that all staff are part of the health care process
Patients should know who all staff are, so that they can talk to the right person. One way of doing this is by the reception staff having a uniform and everyone wearing name badges. There could also be a board in the waiting room with named photographs so that patients can recognize who is who and what they do.

The plan needs also to ensure that the part staff play within the team is continually developed and reinforced. They also need clear guidelines regarding the limits of their authority.

5   Staff Training
It is essential that all staff are trained to the right level and that training is continually maintained by the use of refresher courses. In the case of new staff it is crucial that they understand from the outset what is expected of them. All too often, however, the style of many practices is to throw the new starter in at the deep end, in what is very often one of the most critical positions – answering the telephone. Whilst there are always pressures to make sure that staff are productive as quickly as possible, any new employee needs to be trained in the basic procedures before being let loose.

In many cases, the staff who prove most resistant to customer care training are those who have been in the practice the longest, believing that they should not be treated as learners along with the new recruits. However, if you are to achieve a high standard across the practice as a whole, all staff need to be made fully aware of what you are aiming for and what their good and bad behaviour patterns are. Recognizing this, never compromise by giving in to individual members of staff and allowing them to miss out on training sessions. Instead, use them as the basis for team building as well as developing newly focused, customer care skills.

Once the training process is in hand you can plan ways in which effective performance can be highlighted and rewarded. One idea might be 'employee of the month' recognized by a photograph of the member of staff and the title of the award being posted prominently in the waiting room. Remember also that this should not be limited just to, say, the reception staff, but be open to everyone from the part-time cleaner right through to the senior partner.

Stage four: Measuring practice performance

Having set out to develop a customer care programme, you need to monitor progress and performance on a regular basis. At the outset, therefore, you need to identify your ten most important customer care dimensions and then, using the sorts of techniques that we discussed in Chapter four, measure your performance on these on either a monthly or a quarterly basis. You need then to make use of this information by feeding back the good and the bad points to everyone in the practice and, where appropriate, name the sorts of changes that need to be made to get back on target.

In high street retailing, one of the most consistently effective ways of measuring customer care performance has proved to be by means of 'mystery shoppers.' The mystery shopper (MS), who is either an employee from head office or a market researcher, is used by the retailer to explore particular parts of the operation such as the returns policy, the ways in which difficult customers are handled, and the ability of staff to cope with problems at periods of peak demand. The MS therefore goes into the shop, behaves like a customer, and then feeds the details of the experiences, be they good or bad, to head office.

Although we are not making out a case here for mystery patients, there are several lessons that can be learned from this, and in particular the need to take an objectively detailed and, in the real sense of the word, naive look at various parts of the practice *from the patients' point of view.* It is in this way that you can build up a far clearer picture and understanding of what is going right and what is going wrong.

SUMMARY

Within this chapter, we have highlighted the sorts of issues that need to be taken into account in developing a customer/patient care programme within the practice. As with many of the initiatives that we have discussed in earlier chapters, you need to identify clearly what your objectives are and then, having determined how these will be achieved, ensure that there is total commitment from across the practice and that the responsibility for driving the programme forward is clearly allocated. Given this, think about the following questions which are then pulled together in the form of a customer care action plan in Box 10.3.

• Do you handle your customers in a way that you can be proud of?

• As a practice, do you have a clear and agreed view of the sort of customer care policy that would really be appropriate?

• What will you have to do in order to implement this?

- Who will take on the responsibility for driving it?

- Do you put sufficient pressure upon providers such as hospitals to ensure that they also have an effective customer care policy?

Box 10.3:   The customer care action plan

Our customer care policy is:

The weaknesses in our current approach are:

-

-

-

To overcome these weaknesses, we need to take action in the following areas:

Action areas	Timescales	Responsibility
•		
•		
•		

The performance measures that will be used to monitor our progress are:

Performance measures	Responsibility
Monthly	
•	
•	
•	
•	

continued over

Box 10.3:   *continued*

Performance measures   Responsibility

Quarterly

•

•

•

Annually

•

•

•

11

Internal marketing, leadership and teamworking: fighting the Napoleonic complex

Having read this chapter, you should:

- understand what is meant by internal marketing;

- appreciate the significance of the contribution that internal marketing can make to the effective working of the practice;

- recognize the importance of the vision, strategy, leadership para-
  digm;

- have a greater understanding of what contributes to more effective
  teams;

- appreciate some of the issues associated with effective leadership.

A point that we have made at several stages in this book is that often plans either falter or fail because of the difficulties associated with their implementa-tion. Recognition of this has led in recent years to a considerable amount of attention having been paid to the ways in which internal marketing, team building and particular styles of leadership can make the process of implementing a plan both easier and more effective. It is to these three areas that we now turn our attention.

VISION, STRATEGY AND LEADERSHIP

Having worked with a wide variety of organizations over the years, we believe strongly that it is possible to distinguish between good and bad organizations, that is those that are effective and those that are ineffective, by examining them against the background of the deceptively simple model that is illustrated in figure 11.1.

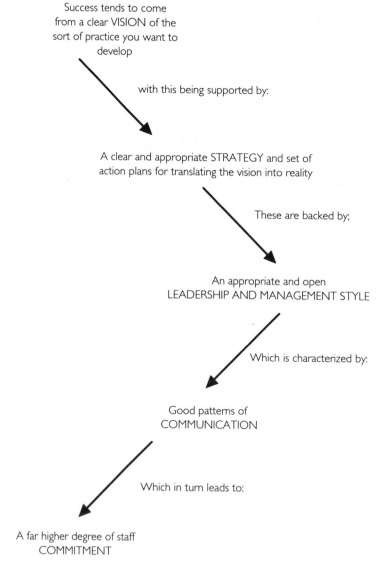

Success tends to come
from a clear VISION of the
sort of practice you want to
develop

with this being supported by:

A clear and appropriate STRATEGY and set of
action plans for translating the vision into reality

These are backed by;

An appropriate and open
LEADERSHIP AND MANAGEMENT STYLE

Which is characterized by:

Good patterns of
COMMUNICATION

Which in turn leads to:

A far higher degree of staff
COMMITMENT

Figure 11.1:   Vision, strategy, leadership . . .

Box 11.1:   The vision, strategy, leadership and communication checklist

The vision

- How clear a vision exists of the sort of practice that you and your partners are trying to develop? (In answering this you might refer back to our discussion of the importance of vision in Chapter seven.)

- To what extent is this vision clouded either by disharmony between the partners or a failure to discuss it in detail?

- Given your location, resources and any other constraints, how realistic is this vision?

- How effectively has this vision been communicated to staff throughout the practice?

The strategy and action plan

- How well thought out are the action plans?

- How explicit are they?

- How well resourced are they?

- How well have patterns of responsibility been allocated?

The leadership/management styles

- What sort of leadership/management style exists within the practice?

- What degree of balance is there between the different styles of the partners?

- How appropriate are these styles, given the sorts of staff that you have and the demands of the late 1990s?

- How do the staff perceive these styles?

- What evidence is there of dissatisfaction among them?

Communication

- How well developed are the patterns of communication within the practice?

- Does information flow in all directions?

- What obstacles to good information flow exists?

- What communication-related problems have been encountered?

The thinking behind the model is straightforward. If an organization, regardless of its type or size, is to move ahead effectively, it is essential that those running it have a clear *vision* of the sort of organization they are trying to develop; that there is a clear *strategy* and set of action plans for achieving this; and that a clear and appropriate *leadership/management* style exists. These are then reinforced by open patterns of *communication* so that the staff are fully aware of the direction in which the organization is going, what is expected of them and how they will benefit. Given this, *levels of commitment* are likely to increase substantially.

To apply the model to your practice, work through the checklist that appears in Box 11.1.

Quite deliberately, we have not asked any questions about levels of commitment. It should be apparent by now that the commitment of staff will be influenced to a very substantial degree by the leadership/management styles and patterns of communication that exist within the practice. However, before going any further and discussing how levels of commitment might be increased by internal marketing, it is worth taking a step sideways and looking at the work of Douglas McGregor in the 1950s and, in particular, his development of the Theory X and Theory Y. In essence, McGregor argues that there are few inherently bad employees, but plenty of bad managers. People, he suggested, typically have the capacity for self-motivation and in general it is the management styles, organizational structures and constraints which inhibit this and prevent them from making a worthwhile contribution; these ideas are summarized in Box 11.2.

It follows from this, and indeed from the earlier part of the chapter, that the practice is likely to work in a far more effective manner if certain broad guidelines are adhered to. An important starting point in this is the development of open patterns of communication with staff being kept fully aware of how the organization is developing. Two immensely valuable tools for this are internal marketing and the development of teams.

SO WHAT IS INTERNAL MARKETING ?

The idea of internal marketing is uncomplicated and based on the idea that an organization will operate far more effectively if its staff have a clear understanding of the core values and objectives and are able to identify with these. To achieve this empathy, there is a need to recruit the appropriate types of people, give

Box 11.2:   McGregor's Theory X and Theory Y

Working in the 1950s, McGregor identified two patterns of thought and assumption about people in organizations.

Theory X argues that people are:

- inherently lazy and work as little as possible

- lack ambition, dislike responsibility and prefer to be led

- self-centred, indifferent to organizational needs, and resistant to change

- gullible and not very bright.

By contrast, theory Y suggests that people:

- are not by nature passive or resistant to organization needs, but have become so as the result of their experiences in organizations

- have an enormous capacity for motivation, development and responsibility, and that structures and systems need to be designed to reflect this and reduce the constraints and level of control.

them a strong sense of identity and operating freedom, and support them with good patterns of communication and open management styles. Assuming this is done properly, the pay-offs can be considerable and are likely to be reflected in far higher levels of motivation and commitment (these ideas were first touched upon in our discussion in Chapter one of the Seven S framework).

In the light of these comments, consider the questions below:

- Do the staff really understand the practice's core values and objectives and empathize with them?

- Do you feel that you really have the right type and blend of staff within the practice?

- Do you spend enough time training staff and equipping them with the skills needed?

- How often are problems caused by poor communications?

- Do your staff feel that they have sufficient operating freedom?

- Are the patterns of communication sufficiently open?

- How involved are your staff in deciding how the practice is run?

On the basis of your answers, think about the sorts of leadership styles that exist within the practice (these are discussed again at a later stage in this chapter in Box 11.4 and Figure 11.2). Are they, for example, essentially a reflection of a 'tells' approach in which having made a decision you and your colleague simply tell the staff what to do, or is it rather more of a 'sells' style in which you sell the idea to others by discussing it in some detail and giving consideration to the implications for them? A third approach is the consultative style where you only make the decision after having discussed the various aspects with those who are involved or who are likely to be affected. Internal marketing gives full recognition to the need to carry staff with you and therefore to the crucial importance of making sure that patterns of communications are as open as possible and that staff feel a strong sense of involvement. Without this, it is likely that you are simply failing to exploit the real potential of the practice team.

THE ROLE OF TEAMS WITHIN THE PRACTICE

As part of the overall process of internal marketing and improving the effectiveness of the practice, you need to give explicit consideration to the scope that exists for teamworking and to the nature of any blocks to teamworking that exist currently. In doing this, you must appreciate that every member of staff is, or should be capable of, making a direct or indirect contribution to the effective treatment of a patient. In making this comment, we are returning to the idea that it is not simply the clinical aspects of the consultation that lead to patients going away satisfied or dissatisfied; the non-clinical elements that surround the consultation, and in particular the practice staff, are often capable of exerting a powerful influence upon patients' perceptions. Recognition of this highlights the significance of teams and teamworking within the practice.

THE PROS AND CONS OF TEAMWORKING

The benefits that can come from teamworking can be substantial and include:

- the support that colleagues can give to individuals so that they can more easily work to their strengths;

- the ways in which teams can build upon the different ideas and skills which individual members of the team posses;

- the ways in which the team can capitalize upon the previous experiences of staff in doing a similar job in different circumstances;

- the discovery of particular skills which in normal circumstances might be hidden, but which frequently emerge when teamworking;

- the ways in which, by ensuring staff familiarize themselves with colleagues' jobs, the practice can avoid an overdependence on individuals, reduce the load on some staff members at times of crisis, and reduce the risk of procedures being carried out differently and incorrectly;

- ensuring that the patients can gain from a better 'experience' in a visit to the practice through a more highly co-ordinated approach;

- a sense of shared purpose and the general levels of synergy that teams can achieve.

There are, of course, some potential dangers of teamworking which can cause problems:

- it can expose the weaknesses of some members of staff and reinforce the egos and position of those members of staff who see themselves as 'experts';

- to be successful, teamworking requires staff to alternate between leading, supporting and sidelines roles and this continual change in relationships can prove difficult for some staff to handle.

However, on balance, the pros of teamwork outweigh any possible cons by a substantial margin and so we should examine how more effective teams can be developed within the practice.

BUILDING MORE EFFECTIVE TEAMS

Only rarely, if ever, is there an opportunity to build a practice team from scratch and in many practices there are relatively infrequent opportunities even to modify practice teams other than peripherally when, for example, someone leaves and you take on someone new. It is possible, however, to make

---

Box 11.3:   The teamworking checklist

- What teams do you have within the practice currently?

- Do you make as much use of teams as you might?

- How well do your teams work?

- What obstacles to better teamworking exist?

- Do you have well balanced teams or do they appear to be dominated by particular individuals?

- What changes would be needed in order to achieve a better balance of skills?

- Do the members of the teams appear to have sufficiently complimentary skills?

- What appear to be the attitudes and levels of motivation of various team members currently? Do they need to be modified in any way? (Do not assume that good working relationships automatically leads to effectiveness. Indeed they can lead to a degree of complacency in which old working practices and conventional wisdoms are never challenged or changed for the better.)

- How are junior staff treated and what roles do they appear to be playing within the teams? Are they simply being tolerated or are real efforts being made by other team members to use their skills and develop their abilities?

---

adjustments by controlling some members of staff, encouraging others in a certain direction and, when recruiting, doing it with a deep-seated understanding of the balances and imbalances that exist within different parts of the practice currently. The sorts of question that can help in this by providing a greater insight to your existing teams, appear in Box 11.3. Remember that when forming or building a team, you need to aim for a blend of strengths, skills, personalities and should avoid building one that simply reinforces the status quo.

SO WHAT CONTRIBUTES TO MORE EFFECTIVE TEAMS?

The guidelines for building more effective teams are relatively straightforward and include:

- ensuring that the team has a distinct and measurable purpose;

- providing constructive feedback on performance;

- varying the team's tasks and responsibilities over time;

- rotating staff on a periodic and planned basis so that new talents and ideas are injected to the team and that the membership and patterns of thinking do not become too incestuous or complacent;

- gradually increasing the degree of autonomy;

- encouraging the team to redefine its responsibilities and tasks.

Against the background of these comments, you should be in a position to answer the following questions:

- Do I trust the members of my team?

- Is there mutual trust?

- Is there mutual respect?

- Is the atmosphere open and supportive?

- Can we handle success and failure?

- Are work loads properly balanced?

- Are the team members loyal to me and/or to the practice and to each other?

- Is there mutual support?

- Can I and other team members express true opinions?

- Do we plan, organize, review and communicate effectively?

- Does everyone feel part of the team?

- Have we got a clear direction and strategy?

ASPECTS OF LEADERSHIP: SUPERMEDICS AND INCOMPETENT MEDDLERS

In 1993, we carried out a study amongst practice managers in an attempt to find out how GPs are viewed by their key staff. The findings led us to suggest that 'the average GP is a poor manager who has appalling communication skills, little real idea of how to plan, fewer ideas of how to motivate staff, and typically adopts an inconsistent and idiosyncratic style of management and leadership.' These conclusions need to be seen against the general background of the work in which we examined the principal roles that doctors are typically expected to perform:

- a *professional carer* role

- a *practice leadership* role

- a *team building* and *team player* role.

Although the majority of practice managers did seem to feel that their doctors carried out the professional carer role fairly well, they proved to be far less complimentary about the extent to which the leadership and team roles were either recognized or performed. It was this that then led us to categorize doctors along the two dimensions that we first introduced in Chapter six (their willingness to manage and their ability to manage) and to label them as supermedics, dangermedics, opt-outs or incompetent meddlers (see Figure 6.2).

BALANCING THE THREE ROLES: THE PROBLEMS OF LEADERSHIP

Despite showing that doctors' medical and professional carer skills were generally (but not invariably) acknowledged by their staff, our research revealed an all too common feeling amongst practice managers that GPs use this as an excuse both for their appalling leadership and team working skills, as well as the way in which staff are frequently expected to operate by telepathy and explain to patients what the doctor really said or meant.

With regard to the *leadership* role that doctors need to perform, our work suggested that interpretations amongst doctors of how best to do this appear to vary enormously. For some, leadership equates with giving orders and telling the staff what to do, with little or no real attempt being made to explain why or how; it was this which led us to suggest that in a surprisingly high number of instances there appeared to be a need for GPs to *fight the Napoleonic complex*. For others, but seemingly a minority, leadership proved to be a far more meaningful activity which involved developing strong and effective communica-

---

Box 11.4:   Leadership styles

- The PROPHET has a vision

- The BARBARIAN is pragmatic, forceful and action orientated

- The BUILDER develops structures

- The EXPLORER develops skills

- The SYNERGIST balances skills and structures

- The ADMINISTRATOR integrates systems to achieve perfect financial and management practice

- The BUREAUCRAT applies tight controls, cuts costs and has no desire to be creative

- The ARISTOCRAT inherits, does no work but upsets the team

---

tion networks, giving emphasis to staff development, and ensuring that everyone understood what was expected of them. For yet others, it was something in which they showed a vague, if amateurish, interest every now and again (generally when they did not appear to have much else to do).

A further area which led to problems of leadership was what we labelled the *isolation ward syndrome*, in which practice managers were denied access to areas of information – particularly financial information – and excluded from any involvement in important decisions. Instead they were simply told the outcome of a planning meeting and then expected to show enormous enthusiasm and total commitment to the process of implementation. Contemplate the sort of overall style that you exhibit and, when you work through Box 11.4, ask yourself what your response reveals about you.

BUILDING AND MOTIVATING PRACTICE TEAMS

The third area we looked at was the *team working* role, in particular how GPs interpret this. All too often it appeared that they failed to recognize the extent of the contribution that they need to make, or indeed the significant amount of time and effort that is involved in building, developing and maintaining effective teams. Instead, they gave the impression either that teams would materialize as if by magic, or that the sole responsibility for team building rests with the practice manager. These problems were then exacerbated by the ways in which the *opt-outs, dangermedics* and *incompetent meddlers* automatically blamed staff for lost files and other problems and rarely, if ever, admitted to their mistakes.

When it came to motivation, doctors evidently performed equally badly, seemingly by working on the basis that staff should not worry because they'll be told when they get it wrong (good staff, it is commonly believed by GPs, never need their egos massaging by being told when they get things right!).

THE NINE DEADLY SINS

Typical of the other mistakes made by doctors and which were highlighted by the study were:

* the failure to recognize that staff have work schedules and deadlines and cannot necessarily always take on extra jobs or work late;

* making decisions for their own benefit without thinking of the consequences for others;

* not agreeing the boundaries of staff responsibility and authority;

* always working on a need-to-know basis;

* persisting with poor communication networks so that mistakes are repeated;

* taking a 'don't bother me, I'm too busy' attitude;

* breaking practice rules and undermining the guidelines laid down by the practice manager;

* not knowing enough about individual members of staff, their aspirations, motivations and limitations;

* requiring some staff to go through the practice manager rather than being able to talk directly to the partners.

You might find it useful to take each of the points in turn and think about the extent to which both yourself and others within the practice may be guilty of these sorts of mistakes. Then think about the consequences for the staff and in particular levels of motivation, morale and team effectiveness.

SUMMARY

We started this chapter off by suggesting that the successful implementation of plans is often hampered by certain styles of leadership and poorly developed and badly managed teams; two elements which highlight the need for a programme of internal as well as external marketing. Recognizing this, you need to reflect on how, if at all, internal marketing is manifested within the practice currently and how an internal marketing programme could be developed or improved. As part of this, give thought also to the nature of the teamworking and leadership styles that exist and to what scope there is for their development and improvement. In the case of leadership styles, Figure 11.2 provides a framework for categorizing the predominant styles, not just of the GPs, but also of others in the practice such as the practice manager, the nurses, the reception staff, the administrative staff, and so on. Given that a participative style is arguably the most appropriate for a professional organization such as a medical practice, you might like to consider whether you appear to have the right mix. If not, identify the sorts of problems this creates and decide what would be involved in changing the balance.

Finally, you need to think about the amount of attention you currently pay to internal marketing and how this might be improved. To help with this, you might go back to the seven questions that we posed earlier in the chapter in our explanation of what internal marketing involves, and then consider how you perform in terms of what we refer to as 'the door exercise'. This is a straightforward concept and based on the idea that, like a door, management styles can be open, closed or ajar. In the case of the open door styles, staff make regular and significant contributions to the development of the practice, because they know:

- how the practice works;

- what is expected of them in terms of daily routines;

- how their ideas and suggestions will be evaluated and used;

- what the future aims and objectives of the practice are and how they can contribute;

- that they would be involved if painful decisions had to be made, so they would not come as a bolt out of the blue.

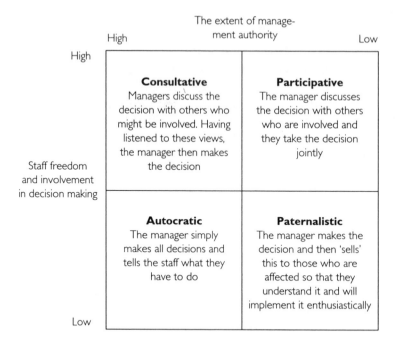

Figure 11.2   The four leadership/management styles

In practices where the door is partially open, staff are kept informed on an irregular basis which is influenced as much by crises and mistakes as anything else. Other stimuli are one of the partners reading a book which advocates open communication and one of the partners needing the staff to rally round when problems arise.

In many ways, this is the worst situation for staff as they never really know where they stand. One day they feel motivated and enthusiastic because their contributions have been asked for and recognized, whilst the next day they will feel ignored and insignificant. In this situation, staff are often expected to offer instant solutions to problems when crises occur, but are not expected to contribute to planning for longer-term improvements and never really know if their unsolicited contributions will be welcome or scorned and do not really know what is expected of them.

Where the door is fully closed, the partners make every decision themselves and let staff have the minimum information that they need to perform their tasks.

The staff in this situation are very clear about their role and what is expected of them. For some, who have no real commitment to the practice, their job is simply a way of earning a salary until they find something better. For others, who look for more from a job, the experience is extraordinarily frustrating. Frequently, these staff feel resentful when their intelligence is insulted and their self-respect is damaged. The partners make it obvious that they have the responsibility for every detail of the practice and as the complexity of running general practice increases, more and more problems emerge. In these circumstances staff retreat, will avoid seeing things that are going wrong and may even feel some satisfaction when a crisis occurs and a partner makes a mistake.

12

Implementing the plan and making things happen

> Having read this chapter, you should:
>
> • understand more clearly the nature and causes of the sorts of factors that help or hinder the development and implementation of marketing plans;
>
> • have a greater insight to the ways in which obstacles might possibly be overcome;
>
> • have developed a framework for implementing a marketing programme for your practice.

Throughout this book, we have concentrated upon developing a relatively pragmatic approach which reflects an emphasis upon the sorts of issues that are associated with the development and implementation of a stronger patient-centred approach to the marketing of general practice. Within this chapter we pull some of these ideas together in the form of an action plan which should provide the framework for your practice's future marketing effort.

THE BARRIERS TO IMPLEMENTATION

On several occasions we have made the observation that planning is generally a relatively straightforward activity, but that numerous plans founder during their implementation. Although there are many reasons for this, the most common have proved to be over-ambitious objectives, unrealistic timescales, inadequate funding, a lack of staff (and partner) commitment and feeling of ownership to its implementation, and, perhaps most importantly, the absence of someone with sufficient authority who is willing to take on the responsibility for driving the plan on a day-to-day basis. Given these points, try to answer the questions below.

- Are you at all guilty of setting objectives that whilst they look impressive, are likely to prove too ambitious?

- Are you trying to do too much in too short a time?

- Have you really thought through the funding implications of the plan and are you confident that funding will not be a problem?

- Are you likely to experience any skills shortages during the period covered by the plan?

- Have you made sure that staff throughout the practice have been involved in the planning process, kept informed of what you are setting out to achieve, and are fully committed to the plan?

- Are *all* the partners fully committed to the plan?

- Have you allocated responsibilities properly?

- Do you have the right person to drive the plan forward (the plan's 'champion')?

- Have you built in the appropriate checks?

- Have you scheduled a series of planning review meetings to monitor progress?

- Have you given sufficient thought to the sorts of factors that might make the implementation of the plan easier and/or more effective?

Assuming that you are satisfied with the answers to these questions, you can then turn your attention to the action-planning framework that is illustrated in Box 12.1; all that remains for us is to wish you happy (and successful) marketing planning!

Box 12.1:   The marketing action-planning framework

Marketing objectives (in order of priority)	Actions required	Timing	Costs	Responsibility	Interim performance measures
•					
•					
•					
•					
•					
•					

13

The Psalter Lane Surgery

The Psalter Lane Surgery is situated in an East Midlands town of some 45,000 people. The town's population is expected to grow by around 15 percent over the next few years. The practice was established in 1935 and has four GPs, each of whom has, until recently, had a full list. Quite deliberately, the partners have developed or been recruited for their complementary skills, something which they believe represents a fundamental strength of the practice. The somewhat autocratic senior partner, Dr Michael Harrison, is the practice's expert in paediatrics, whilst the others have special interests in geriatrics (Dr Vanessa Grant), asthma and diabetes (Dr Faheem Jaiswal), and gynaecology and general medicine (Dr Tom McDonald). The ages of the partners are 62, 64, 53, and 32 respectively.

The doctors are supported by two Sisters who are responsible for nursing care, a number of the specialist clinics, and innoculations. The administration is in the hands of a 64-year-old senior receptionist who has two full-time and three part-time receptionists to help her and who she rules with a rod of iron. Surgery hours are as follows:

Doctors	08.00–11.00	Monday–Friday
	17.00–19.00	
	09.00–10.30	Saturday
Sisters	08.15–12.15	Monday–Friday
	14.30–19.00	

The surgery is based in a converted, turn of the century building which is increasingly proving to be cramped and old-fashioned. Behind the building are parking spaces for six cars, all of which are reserved for the medical staff. The nearest public car park is 300 metres away but, because of its proximity to the town centre, this is often full. A bus route passes the surgery door and there is a bus stop 50 metres away.

The building's ground floor consists of a reception and waiting area and three of the four surgeries. The fourth surgery, together with the Sisters' surgery and the toilets, are on the first floor. The reception staff work from behind a chest-high counter. Having reported to reception, patients sit in the waiting area until their doctor is free; this is announced by a flashing light, a buzzer and the receptionist calling out the name of the patient.

Patients' records are detailed and the system is tightly controlled, with all files that have been used by the partners or staff having to be accounted for at the end of each surgery period. The telephone system was last updated five years ago and, with too few lines, is increasingly being found to be inadequate, with the result that it is often difficult to make an external call. Equally, patients frequently find the lines engaged when trying to make an appointment. Outside surgery hours, a medical deputizing service is used for emergencies.

A rival practice is based a mile away in a new purpose-built building. Its three partners have developed a strong reputation for their levels of patient care and up-to-date approach. Because of this, the Psalter Lane Surgery has recently lost a number of its younger patients.

The youngest of the Psalter Lane's partners, Tom McDonald has recently expressed a number of concerns to the others and has suggested that unless a more proactive stance is adopted, it seems likely that the practice will continue to suffer a decline. As evidence of this, he highlighted the loss of patients to the rival practice, the increased number of complaints from patients in recent months, and the limited number of specialist clinics offered by the practice. Recognition of the possible validity of McDonald's argument has lead to the partners having agreed to him conducting a detailed review of the practice.

To help with this, he turned to a copy of *Marketing and General Practice* by Colin Gilligan and Robin Lowe that had recently arrived on his desk. As he leafed through the book, his ideas began to crystallize. He thought in detail about each of the elements of the practice's marketing mix and began drawing up his results shown in Box 13.1.

Looking at the comments that he had jotted down, McDonald's heart sank as he began to recognize the extent to which the practice would have to change if it was to become truly patient-centred. He then turned back to the book and flipped through the pages almost at random, stopping only to note down a few of the questions that seemed to spring off the page. Included in these were those in Chapter one:

Box 13.1: Tom McDonald's initial evaluation of the practice's marketing mix

Product

Positive
- A range of specialist medical services;
- A well-established, albeit rather old-fashioned, reputation for sound no-nonsense medical advice.

Negative
- An appoinments' system that reflects the doctors' needs and preferences rather than those of the patients;
- Cover out of hours via a medical answering services;
- A down at heel waiting room that features a variety of different types of chair, some out of date (and torn) magazines, several broken toys and an ill-fitting carpet;
- A rather abrupt system of calling patients;
- Surgeries for the Sisters and one for the doctors are on the first floor;
- Toilets which are also on the first floor;
- Car parking which is totally inadequate.

Place/physical aspects

Positive
- Nothing obvious.

Negative
- Poor location with inadequate parking;
- Poorly equipped and old-fashioned building;
- Home visits by a medical deputizing service;
- The area surrounding the practice is beginning to look rather run down;
- Notice board with out-of-date and peeling notices.

continued over

Box 13.1:   *continued*

Promotion

Positive	**Negative**
• Nothing obvious.	• A very amateurish practice leaflet that has been printed on poor paper; • No practice newsletter.

Price

McDonald recognized the particular problems of analysing the price component of general practice and concentrated upon producing a list of questions to which he felt that he needed answers:

- What funds for expansion could we lay our hands on?
- Is our profit level as high as it might be?
- Are we exploiting all possible sources of income?
- Do we send invoices out on time?
- Do we chase payment of these?
- Are we paying creditors on time?
- What is our cash flow like?
- How cost-effective are we?
- What costs are associated with each major dimension of the practice?
- In what areas are costs too high?
- What would be the costs and revenues associated with a series of new clinics?

People

Positive	**Negative**
• Highly committed senior receptionist;	• Poor people management skills on the part of the senior receptionist;
• Highly committed and skilled nursing staff;	• No real commitment to staff training;
• Strong medical skills amongst the doctors.	• Traditional and rather formal patterns of communication;
	• Too high a rate of turnover amongst the junior reception staff.

continued opposite

Box 13.1:   *continued*

Proccess management

Positive	Negative
• The senior receptionist ensures the system works smoothly;	• Inadequate computerization;
• An accurate system of records.	• A rather abrupt system of calling patients.

- To what extent have the challenges facing general practice been given explicit recognition?

- What specific plans exist to deal with them?

- Has the responsibility for dealing with these challenges been allocated?

The answers he realized were 'not at all,' 'none,' and 'no.'

Turning to Box 1.3, he gave the practice a total score of 13, the absolute minimum. In the case of Box 1.4, the results were very similar. And so it went on. Looking at Chapter five, he realized that he and his partners were classic examples of boiled frogs, something which was in turn reflected in Box 5.2 and the uncannily accurate description of the first of the four types of practice. Looking at Figure 5.4, he saw how the description of the practice ostriches applied almost perfectly.

Faced with this, he put the book down and sat back. What we need, he thought, is an action plan, something which help us to face up to some of the challenges and capitalize upon the opportunities. Fired with enthusiasm, he turned back to the book and began listing some of the activities and tools that would be of help, including:

- a survey of patients so that he and his partners could understand more fully how the practice was perceived (Chapter four);

- a more detailed SWOT analysis, with attention being paid to the conversion of weaknesses into strengths and threats into opportunities (Box 7.2, Figure 7.2 and Chapter eight);

- a programme of internal marketing (Chapter eleven);

- the Ansoff matrix (Figure 9.3);

- areas of patient need and levels of funding support (Box 9.2 and Figure 9.4).

Although this was by no means an exhaustive list, he recognized that it provided a useful starting point. As the building quietened and the lights went out as the staff left for the evening (it was five past seven, after all), he began his first attempt at completing the Ansoff matrix . . . (see Figure 13.1).

Product/services

	Current	New
Current	• Achievement of targets for vaccinations and cervical cytology • Primary care medical services	• Recruitment of a new partner with a specialty • Well man/well woman • Stress management • Bereavement counselling • Sports injury advice • Minor surgical procedures
New	• Well man/well woman • Sports injury advice • Satellite surgery to attract new patients	• Promotion of the new partner's skills into new sectors

Markets (row label, between Current and New)

Figure 13.1   Tom McDonald's first attempt at the Ansoff matrix

Index